BEEF BUSTERS

BEEF BUSTERS

Marissa Cloutier M.S., R.D.
with Deborah S. Romaine
and Eve Adamson

Produced by Amaranth

ADAMS MEDIA CORPORATION
Avon, Massachusetts

Published by
Adams Media Corporation
57 Littlefield Street, Avon, MA 02322 U.S.A.
www.adamsmedia.com

Produced by
Amaranth
Oxford, MD

Design by RB Design New York, NY
Printed in Canada.

ISBN: 1-58062-638-6

J I H G F E D C B A

Library of Congress Cataloging-in-Publication data available
upon request from the publisher.

This publication is designed to provide accurate and authoritative information with
regard to the subject matter covered. It is sold with the understanding that the publisher is not engaged in rendering legal, accounting, or other professional advice. If
legal advice or other expert assistance is required, the services of a competent professional person should be sought.

> —From a *Declaration of Principles* jointly adopted by a
> Committee of the American Bar Association and
> a Committee of Publishers and Associations

This book is available at quantity discounts for bulk purchases.
For information, call 1-800-872-5627.

This book is dedicated to beef-loving Beef Busters everywhere.
Although you probably haven't met a steak you didn't like,
we hope you bust beef from your diet with the help of this book.

Contents

Foreword

As a health inspector for a local health department, I observe food handling at the retail level, somewhere near the end of the path stretching from farm to table. There are plenty of things that can go wrong, both in food establishments' handling of food and in the transportation, storage, and preparation by the consumer—improper temperatures, cross-contamination by way of raw food products, dirty wiping rags, improper hand washing, unsanitized equipment, sneezes . . . the list goes on. If it happens in the retail setting, or, for that matter, wholesale setting, it surely has the potential to occur in home kitchens. Retailers and wholesalers have regulations to follow to help ensure food safety, but once the food is home, it is up to you, the consumer, to handle it safely.

The United States is believed to have the safest food supply in the world. It is a sad fact of life, however, that the foods on which we rely for sustenance are capable of causing or transmitting illness, and even death. The Centers for Disease Control and Prevention (CDC) have estimated that food-borne illnesses are responsible for thousands of deaths in the United States each year, and millions of people annually will suffer from illnesses stemming from food-borne pathogens (disease-producing organisms).

In the last decade, the public has become more aware of the risks involved in food safety, even if they are unable to match the pathogen with the associated food product(s). Highly publicized outbreaks of food poisoning from *Escherichia coli* O157:H7 and *Listeria monocyto-genes*, among others, have contributed to this heightened awareness. *Salmonella enteriditis* helped make New Jersey the butt of a late night talk show joke when it looked like health officials would be busting people for serving runny eggs at the local diner. Now, even when entering the local supermarket, consumers can't help but get the message about food safety. Food packages have labels detailing safe handling procedures and many supermarket chains have brochures available to promote food safety awareness.

You do have choices, though, and in making a choice, safety is sometimes sacrificed. It is important to know the risks involved when choosing to eat those eggs over easy or a rare hamburger. Risks are also taken when choosing food, from a nutritional standpoint. Most consumers are now familiar with the USDA food pyramid, and with the daily servings it recommends. Yet many people do not follow these nutritional guidelines, potentially leading to chronic diseases.

As you read this book, you will learn about choices—choices associated with beef consumption. You may already know how to cook hamburgers to reduce the risk of food poisoning from *Escherichia coli* O157:H7, but there are other compelling reasons to examine beef consumption. While there is no evidence at this time of its existence in the United States, bovine spongiform encephalopathy (BSE), commonly known as mad cow disease, has spread through cattle herds in Europe. New variant Creutzfeldt-Jakob disease (vCJD) is believed to be its human equivalent; vCJD is thought to be caused by the same kind of agent that causes BSE—a protein substance known as a "prion." Unlike *E. coli* O157:H7, this is not something that can be eliminated by cooking.

Eating safely and eating for health really are two different goals, but they do have one thing in common: Choice. Make informed choices; do the right thing for your health and for your safety.

—NANCY A. TARANTINO, M.S.
   Registered Environmental Health Specialist and Health Officer,
   New Jersey Health Department

Introduction

Are you sure that the beef you are feeding your family is 100 percent safe? It seems that we are bombarded with a steady stream of recalls for food-borne pathogens such as *Salmonella, Listeria monocytogenes,* and *Escherichia coli* O157:H7. But at least these pathogens can be identified, contained, and destroyed through proper processing and cooking methods. There is a new and dangerous threat lurking within one of the Western world's favorite foods. One that is not so easily identified, contained, or destroyed.

What if something you ate today could cause your slow, agonizing death years or even decades from now? Would knowing that this food was a potential time bomb, seeding your body with the agents of its eventual destruction, be enough to cause you to give up this food? It seems that every time you open a newspaper or turn on the evening news, there are reports of studies linking foods to health consequences, including heart disease and cancer. Indeed, there have been many warnings in recent decades of the hazards of the modern Western diet and lifestyle. So many, in fact, that a lot of people are tempted just to tune out.

It is time to pay attention.

The Unique and Terrifying Specter of Mad Cow Disease

One of the most horrifying threats is the emergence of a so-far rare but fatal disease popularly referred to as mad cow disease. Scientists call this disease bovine spongiform encephalopathy (BSE). It eats holes in the brains of infected cows, causing them to behave as though crazed. And in people who eat meat from infected cows, BSE can cause a human form of the disease called variant Creutzfeldt-Jakob disease (vCJD).

This human form of mad cow disease creates spongelike pockets in the brain as it slowly destroys brain tissue, putting its victims through unspeakable mental and physical anguish for the two years or so that they survive after the onset of symptoms. There is no treatment to mitigate those symptoms, which include personality changes, paranoia, and loss of bodily movements and functions. And there is no cure. The mother of a nineteen-year-old French boy, one of a handful of vCJD victims in France, told the news-reporting agency Reuters, "He died in appalling conditions. He looked like an old man."

Variant Creutzfeldt-Jakob disease claimed 100 lives in Europe (mostly in Britain), where the disease first surfaced, between 1996 and 2001. While this seems a small number compared to the thousands of people who die every day as a result of heart disease or cancer, many health officials fear the worst is yet to come. "Beef is one of the great unifying symbols of our culture," wrote the British newspaper *The Guardian* in a 1996 editorial. "The Roast Beef of Old England is a fetish, a household god, which has suddenly been revealed as a Trojan horse for our destruction." The United Nations has issued an international call to nations to act swiftly to prevent the spread of mad cow disease throughout the world.

Europeans are eating barely two-thirds as much beef as they consumed before the BSE crisis, and now it seems that Americans might be following suit. A March 2001 Gallup poll revealed that seven in ten Americans are worried about mad cow disease, and as a result one-quarter of Americans have cut back on the amount of meat they eat or have stopped eating meat altogether.

While health experts agree that no one yet knows the full extent of the BSE/vCJD crisis, many are concerned that consuming contaminated beef products has exposed potentially millions of people. It took 10 years for British officials to recognize the seriousness of BSE and to implement measures designed to curtail its spread. It is possible that in those 10 years infected beef products, feed products, and live cattle made it to markets around the world.

BSE can take as long as eight years to develop in cattle, during which time diseased animals show no symptoms; and most cattle are slaughtered when they are three or four years old. Unless scientists examine its brain (a costly and time-consuming process), there is no way to know whether a cow has the brain-wasting disease. To counter this, Britain (where the disease first showed up) has slaughtered millions of cattle as a precautionary measure and prohibits the use of meat or other products from any animal over 30 months old unless the animal's brain tests negative for BSE.

Variant Creutzfeldt-Jakob disease, the human form of mad cow disease, takes even longer to show itself in people who become infected. So far, vCJD seems to take about 10 years to begin causing symptoms. Some scientists believe the incubation period could be even longer, up to 20 years or more. In a September 1998 article in *The Atlantic Monthly*, researcher Stephen Morse likened the potential of vCJD to the AIDS epidemic, pointing out that in the beginning scientists throughout the world underestimated the likely consequences of what looked like a rare disease that subsequently became a widespread and devastating crisis that health officials have yet to be able to curb.

In the article, Morse noted that while vCJD doesn't appear to spread as easily as HIV, the virus that causes AIDS, it does seem able to exist in the body for a long time without causing any signs of disease. More worrisome, however, are mistakes health officials made when knowledge of the relationship between BSE and vCJD was limited—a time when, unfortunately, a significant level of infection might have already taken place, which we might not learn about for years to come.

Modern Processing Methods Spread Mad Cow Disease through Europe

A British veterinarian saw the first known case of mad cow disease in 1986, on a farm in southern England. At the time, no one had ever seen such an ailment. Although the farmer lost nine cows to the bizarre condition, neither he nor the veterinarian suspected the deaths were the start of a crisis that would virtually decimate the British cattle industry. Six years later, when veterinary officials realized that they had an epidemic on their hands, nearly 200,000 cattle had already died from what scientists finally identified as BSE. Faced with the likelihood that hundreds of thousands of other cattle could be infected, the British government ordered millions of cattle killed in a desperate effort to halt the disease's spread. Most health experts now agree that it was too little, much too late.

Scientists suspect modern processing methods shoulder significant blame for the spread of BSE—not because these methods are faulty, but because they have become so efficient. As far back as the 1930s, cattle farmers realized they could get more meat from their cows if they fed them a diet high in protein. And it wasn't much of a leap to further realize that they had an inexpensive form of protein right under their noses: the waste from slaughtered cattle. After processing at extreme temperatures, rendered animal protein (the boiled-down remains of carcasses) was added to animal feed products called meat and bone meal (MBM) feeds.

In 1988, when it became clear that the remains of cattle with BSE were certainly included in MBM feeds, Britain banned its farmers from feeding MBM products to their cattle. But the ban did not cover feeding MBM to other animals such as poultry and pigs, and it did not cover exports. So manufacturers continued to make MBM feed products for other livestock. Feed manufacturers also continued making

MBM cattle feed for export to other countries, selling millions of tons of potentially contaminated feed to cattle farmers throughout the world over the following eight years.

By 1996, British health officials realized that cross-contamination among feed products was rampant. MBM managed to find its way into feed that British farmers believed was MBM-free, causing at least 60,000 more cases of BSE before the British government totally banned the manufacture and use of MBM feed products. Unfortunately, only time will tell whether the complete ban came quickly enough. With BSE-contaminated MBM feed products feeding millions of cattle throughout Europe and Southeast Asia, it could be another five to ten years before health officials know what role the exported products played in extending the range and incidence of BSE infections in cattle and corresponding vCJD infections in people.

Europe Prepares for Round Two

Even as U.S. health officials are rushing to reassure the American public that BSE does not exist on American soil, European countries are struggling with a second wave of mad cow disease as scientists confirm cases of BSE in cattle in the Czech Republic. "It's the first caused by re-exports," microbiologist Dr. Stephen Dealler told Reuters in a June 2001 interview. "We are seeing a potential indicator that the epidemic in Europe is greater than was expected."

What this means is that while nearly all cases of BSE in cattle identified between 1994 and 2000 could be traced to cows imported directly from Britain (including one that made it to Canada), the new cases that are cropping up are being traced to cattle exported from countries such as Germany and France. These are cattle that have no connection to Britain. Scientists aren't entirely certain how these cattle contracted BSE, but suspect it was through MBM feed.

German health officials expect to see at least 500 new cases of BSE in 2001, after several years of assuring the German public that mad cow disease was not a problem in Germany. Renate Keunast, Germany's agriculture minister, told PBS's Paul Miller in an interview for Online NewsHour in January 2001, "We are not at the end of fighting against BSE; we are somewhere in the middle."

A Worldwide Risk

The World Health Organization (WHO) continues to raise concerns about the potential spread of BSE and vCJD, fearing that lax import and export restrictions in less-affluent countries will allow the diseases to gain footholds in new territories. After a joint conference on BSE in June 2001, which brought together more than 150 veterinarians, food safety experts, and health officials for a four-day summit in Paris, WHO issued a strident warning:

> Bovine Spongiform Encephalopathy (BSE) and variant Creutzfeldt-Jakob Disease (vCJD) should be considered an international issue as materials potentially infected with BSE have been distributed throughout the world through trade in live cattle, certain cattle products, and byproducts. All countries are urged to evaluate their potential exposure and should take necessary actions.

The scientists urged all countries to ban MBM feed from use in cattle, sheep, and other ruminants and to establish structured surveillance and testing procedures to detect cattle infected with BSE before they make it to the slaughterhouse.

Are Efforts to Keep Mad Cow Out of the United States Enough?

U.S. health officials believe a series of precautions taken in the United States since the identification of BSE in 1988 and the recognition in 1996 of its correlation to vCJD in people are adequate to ensure that BSE has not infiltrated the American beef industry. But vCJD takes 10 years or longer to show itself. The best-case scenario is that it would be at least 2006 before beef-eating Americans could breathe easy; in practicality, it will be much longer.

While U.S. health officials insist that the American beef supply is safe, world health experts urge greater caution in reaching such a conclusion. Numerous scientists point to the false security health officials in European countries such as Britain, Belgium, France, and Germany had and the reassurances they conveyed to the public about the risks of BSE and vCJD. Numerous politicians in these countries resigned or lost their posts in response to public outcry about their handling of the crisis. Some scientists are concerned that the United States and other countries that consider themselves "safe" are sliding the same slippery slope.

From 1988, when British veterinarians diagnosed the first cases of BSE in cattle, until 1996, when the first cases of vCJD were diagnosed in people, Britain followed the same restrictions on beef by-products in animal feed that are now in place in the United States. And in the beginning, the British government took pretty much the same posture about the safety of British beef as the American government is now taking about the safety of American beef. Officials believed that because they saw no signs of illness in humans, BSE was a disease confined to cattle. By the time it became clear that this was not the case, the consequences were tragic.

In some ways, however, it appears that the American government learned from its European counterparts. The U.S. Department of Agriculture (USDA) banned MBM feeds imported from Britain in 1988, an action many experts credit with keeping BSE out of the American beef supply at a time when it was infiltrating cattle herds throughout Europe. But other experts aren't so sure of the effort's success, citing the extensive incubation periods for both BSE and vCJD. It is far too early, some scientists believe, to feel confident about anything when it comes to these diseases.

One ongoing concern is incomplete compliance with MBM feed restrictions. Although the Food and Drug Administration (FDA) and USDA banned feeding MBM to cattle, these products remain available and are popular for feeding to other animals. This establishes a fairly high risk for cross-contamination of feed products intended for cattle—a problem that many scientists believe allowed the BSE crisis to explode in Britain. And as recently as January 2001, an FDA study found some American feed manufacturers were still using bone meal and rendered animal protein in feed products that were being fed to cattle, including one incident in which 22 tons of MBM-contaminated feed products were recalled and 1,200 cattle were quarantined after eating the feed suspected to be tainted.

Nor does the United States have a structured surveillance and testing program in place—at least not one that satisfies international standards. Of particular concern is the practice of examining the brains of only "downers"—cattle that are killed because they go down or become unable to walk for some, often unknown, reason. USDA officials point out that as of June 2001, no tested cattle brains have come back positive for BSE; critics counter that cattle infected with BSE will often show no symptoms.

Consumer advocacy groups are calling for stricter federal policies on testing standards and monitoring programs for BSE in the United States, asserting that the USDA can do more to ensure that mad cow disease is not present here in the United States. A recent editorial in the *New England Journal of Medicine* also asked for greater federal scrutiny.

Most European countries test far more cattle than are tested in the United States. In 10 years of random testing for BSE, the USDA has examined the brains of 12,000 cattle and found no evidence of BSE—yet on average there are about 180,000 downers each year. In Western Europe, by comparison, government veterinarians test *every* downer. Unlike in the United States, where downers can find their way into rendering plants, farmers in countries such as Britain and France cannot destroy or dispose of any cattle that die before slaughter until they have been tested for BSE.

As well, there are concerns that the American practice of slaughtering cattle by shooting them in the heads with pneumatic stun guns (devices that deliver a lethal force of air pressure) before slitting their throats, might be exchanging expediency and perceived humanity for increased risk. The method can blow brain tissue into other parts of the cow's body (inspectors have found brain tissue in a cow's lungs and liver).

All eyes are on the USDA as the U.S. policy on mad cow disease continues to evolve. The stakes are high as citizens, from home cooks to food experts, look for assurances that U.S. beef is safe. When asked by *USA Weekend* about worries over mad cow disease, popular Food Network chef and restaurant owner Mario Batali voiced the common concern of many Americans, "I don't know answers to all the questions [about safety]. But I'm not willing to bet my grandkids' legs on them. I'm very worried about it, and I hope the USDA will do the right thing. They'd better."

The Economic Effects of BSE

Since 1988, health officials in Europe have destroyed millions of cattle, mostly in Britain. Though the rate of infection has slowed especially in Britain, most countries that belong to the European Union have adopted the practice of killing all cattle in a herd when one cow is diagnosed with BSE. With people buying half as much beef as before the BSE crisis, farmers who have healthy herds of cattle are seeing the bottom drop out of the beef market. Because many countries around the world refuse to accept beef and beef products from countries where BSE is known to exist (or sometimes even suspected to exist), there is little demand for European-grown beef. Limits on beef products intended to reduce the risk of BSE-infected meat getting into the food supply have also increased both waste and manufacturing costs. Economic losses already extend well into the billions (of American dollars) and continue to climb.

There is a silver lining of sorts to the depressed European beef market for American beef manufacturers, who have seen exports of beef products to Europe rise more than a third. Beef from the United States is considered BSE-free because there has not yet been a case of BSE identified in the country, making it eligible for import into European Union member nations.

Taking Appropriate Precautions

Although cooking to proper temperatures kills the pathogens that cause other food-borne infections, it appears to have little if any effect on the infectious agent that causes BSE and vCJD. Scientists consider all meat from an infected cow to be capable of carrying the infectious agent, although most researchers believe the infectious prions that cause BSE concentrate in brain and spinal cord tissues. These tissues are among the beef by-products banned in many countries. Health officials believe muscle meats such as steaks and roasts are least likely to carry BSE infection; ground meats such as hamburger and sausage are the most likely to carry BSE infection since they can contain fragments of brain or nerve tissue.

Health officials at the Centers for Disease Control and Prevention (CDC) recommend that Americans traveling to Europe, and other parts of the world, such as Southeast Asia, where BSE is a known or potential problem take these precautions:

- Choose to eat foods other than beef.
- If you choose to eat beef, select muscle meat such as steak or roast that is certified BSE-free.
- Avoid ground beef (hamburger) and sausage.

WHO standards consider a country or region to be BSE-free only when there have been no identified cases of BSE in cattle for at least seven years. Every time a new case is diagnosed, the countdown begins anew. In July 2001, Britain was still recording about 30 new cases of BSE a week—and Greece reported its first case. It will be a long time, if ever, that any country in the world can consider itself free from the risk of BSE and vCJD.

Living Beef-Free

No matter how worried you might be about diseases such as mad cow and vCJD, the risk of *Escherichia coli* O157:H7 infection or other food-borne illnesses, or the risk of heart disease or cancer, it isn't always easy to change a lifetime of beef-eating habits. It's okay that you like beef; it's been what's for dinner for decades. But it's also great that you recognize the need to cut back on the beef you eat or even eliminate it entirely from your diet. There's much we haven't known about beef until recent years, so the time is right to make the changes that are best for your lifestyle and your health.

Maybe you've been gradually shifting away from beef, and now recognize that you are ready to make the move official. Perhaps reading this book will confirm your decision to live beef-free. So to help you keep moving on your journey of change to a vital beef-free lifestyle, we've organized the Beef Buster plan for healthy eating into four steps:

Reduce. Is there too much beef in that bun? Many people eat larger portions of beef than they realize. The first step in busting beef from your diet is to identify how much beef you are eating in one sitting and begin to eat smaller portion sizes. Because you also want to reduce the amount of saturated fat that you're eating, another element of reducing is to choose leaner cuts of meat. You'll also want to start eliminating ground beef and sausage products from your diet, which have been linked most strongly in Europe to BSE-contamination as they are more likely to contain pieces of spinal or brain tissues.

Substitute. Many people eat beef more often than they realize. If you're eating beef "eight days a week," that's about seven days too many! The second step in busting free from beef is to find other, often more nutritious, meats and foods that can begin replacing beef in your diet.

Incorporate. Once you're not eating all that beef, you'll discover a vast and tasty array of foods that haven't been among your menu choices. At this step, you'll find that eating less beef leaves you more room in your appetite for plant-based foods such as fruits, vegetables, and whole grains that are satisfyingly filling as well as nutritious.

Eliminate. Where's the beef? Who cares! By the time you reach this final step, you might be wondering what all the fuss was about. You'll be eating such a rich and delicious variety of foods, how could you possibly feel that you're missing out by leaving out the beef?

Of course, if you have any medical conditions, you should consult with your doctor before undertaking any changes in your diet. A registered dietitian can provide you with specific recommendations for your medical condition.

You'll want to be on the lookout, as well, for beef by-products in supplements and other processed food products. When in doubt about the safety of any supplement, treatment, or additive, steer clear!

We wish you the best of luck as you endeavor to educate yourself on food safety issues to make sure that the food you put on your family's table is safe, healthfully prepared, and optimally nutritious.

Nutritional Content Sources Cited in This Book

There are many sources for nutritional content of various foods. The nutritional information cited in Chapters 1 through 12 comes from *Bowes & Church's Food Values of Portions Commonly Used*, 17th ed., by Jean A. Pennington (Philadelphia: Lippincott-Raven, 1998). The nutritional information for the recipes was calculated using ESHA Research's computerized nutrition analysis software *The Food Processor*.

BEEF
BUSTERS

1

Americans, Beef, and the Wild, Wild West

Americans and beef. The two just go together, like steak and potatoes, burgers and fries, hot dogs and cold soda pop. Every day, we consume more than 77 million servings of beef for a total of about 64 pounds of beef per year per person. In the next two weeks, more than 230 million of us (more than 90 percent of American households) will eat beef at least one meal—for 80 percent of us it'll be at dinner; for 17 percent, at lunch. Nearly 20 percent will eat steaks, whereas another 12 percent will have burgers. Steaks and burgers top the popularity list when dining out, too. Americans eat more than 360 million steaks and nearly 6 billion burgers in restaurants each year. This compares to 5 billion servings of chicken, 2 billion servings of seafood, and 500 million servings of pork. Will Americans keep their love affair with beef at any cost? Just how did this love affair begin, and what keeps it going so strong? The answer starts back . . . way back . . . in history.

In the Beginning . . . Not Quite Beef as We Know It

Most anthropologists believe humans have been meat eaters since the beginning of human existence, a belief supported by evidence at excavated sites in various locations throughout the world that reveal bones, primitive weapons, and other apparent remnants of the hunt. Early humans apparently hunted a variety of animals, from the enormous woolly mammoth to smaller creatures such as the ancestors of modern rabbits, pigs, and birds. Meat was a source of nutrition that helped support the on-the-go nomadic lifestyle of prehistoric hunting-gathering populations.

The meat early humans did eat came from active, wild game not from pen-raised animals fattened before slaughter to ensure well-marbled, tender flesh. This meat might have been red, but it was much lower in saturated fat than the meat we eat today and probably even contained some omega-3 fatty acids, like the "good" heart-healthy fat found in fish. Scientists believe the red meat of this ancient time was more like today's skinless chicken breast than like today's beef in terms of its fat content. Modern farm-raised beef likely contains up to seven times as much saturated fat as did the free-range meat our prehistoric ancestors ate.

Archaeological evidence suggests that early humans weren't purely carnivorous; it appears they also ate wild fruits (such as berries), wild grains, vegetables, nuts, and seeds. Some researchers believe that the prehistoric diet was higher in vegetation than in meat and propose that ancient humans, in fact, ate a largely vegetarian diet. Because so much of their diet came from vegetation, ancient humans could have consumed up to 100 grams of fiber a day. Compare that to the typical American's fiber intake of about 15 grams a day!

Cattle Come to the New World

When the first European explorers landed on the North American continent in the mid-1400s, domesticated cattle farming was well established in most regions of Europe. But in the New World, buffalo, not cattle, grazed the vast plains and grasslands, from the Pacific Ocean to the Eastern Seaboard. Historians believe there were as many as 30 to 75 million of these lumbering beasts, also called bison (their scientific name), roaming in herds that contained hundreds of thousands of animals, before Spanish explorers brought the longhorn cattle to the

Americas in the 1490s. An exceptionally sturdy breed, the longhorn quickly multiplied. Other explorers and settlers brought different breeds of cattle with them, along with sheep, goats, and pigs.

Home on the Range: The American West

It's America's mythology: the cowboy, the steer, and the open range. But for those who lived in the Wild West, life was anything but mythical. Between 1860 and 1890, cattle trails, not paved interstate highways, traversed the rugged terrain of the then-Wild West. Travel was by horse or by horse- or ox-drawn wagon. The routes were hot and dusty in the summers, frigid and windy in the winters. The men (there were very few, if any, women working the herds) who rode the trails bringing cattle to market tolerated a rough, challenging lifestyle. Contrary to legend, few cowmen ("cowboys" were actually boys, usually in their early to mid-teens) enjoyed steak for every meal. The thousands of cattle that they funneled along the trails from the grazing lands to the stockyards were valuable commodities, worth far more to their owners at cattle auctions than the ranchers felt compelled to "pay" the men who drove them. Trail-side meals were more likely to consist of boiled beans seasoned with salt pork than of grilled steaks.

Pioneer families homesteading in the West didn't eat all that much beef, either. Cows provided vital milk, from which settlers could make butter and cheese. Steers were valuable field workers, pulling plows and dragging logs. When a cow or steer did die or had to be slaughtered because of injury, just about every inch and ounce was put to use in some way. Hides, tanned and sometimes dyed, became coats, hats, and gloves. Fat, or tallow, became candles and soap. After eating as much meat as possible (and preserving some cuts in underground ice pits, if ice was available), the hardworking farm families dried and smoked strips of beef to eat as jerky during the winter months. Families also ate jerky while driving cattle on the trails and used it in pemmican (powdered dried beef mixed with beef fat and sometimes berries or dried fruit to form a nutritiously dense paste that could be stored for long periods of time). Narrow strips of intestines, cut, dried, and stretched, became guitar and fiddle strings.

The technology of the late 1870s that made long-term freezing a consistent and reliable method of storage greatly extended the availability of beef both geographically and socioeconomically. Between this development and the growing network of railroads, the traditional cowman soon went the way of the woolly mammoth. Growing numbers of people, many of them new immigrants to this country, pushed into the West to start new lives, turning prairie towns into cities and suburbs and ending the pioneer lifestyle.

The "War Generation" and Beef

As the United States entered the 1900s, beef ruled the table and the American diet. Prosperous middle- and upper-class families enjoyed steaks and roasts for breakfast as well as for lunch and dinner, typically accompanied by some form of potatoes, eggs, breads, and biscuits. Total calories were not such a source of anxiety as they are today. The ideal female figure of the time weighed in at a bountiful 200 pounds—close to 90 pounds more than the average model we see gracing our modern fashion magazines. The considerably heftier male physique of the time sported a belly that defied measurement as a waist. This ideal man was a far cry from the six-pack abs today's buff men crave. The fashionably fat referred to their stylish look as "plump."

Innovations in preparation and storage techniques soon established fast food as part of the American culinary landscape. The first chain hamburger restaurant, White Castle, opened its first outlet in 1921 and sold hamburger sandwiches for a nickel each. Advances in food processing, canning, and freezing further improved the availability and convenience of meat products as well as other food items.

World War I, and even more so World War II, dramatically altered the ways Americans ate. Wartime rationing limited dietary staples such as sugar, eggs, milk, and meat—especially beef, which went largely to feed soldiers in training. In between the two World Wars was the Great

Depression, a time of economic collapse and limitations in nearly every dimension of daily life. Chipped dried beef, minced beef, creamed beef, and stews and soups enhanced with bone ends and beef remnants, including organ meats, helped Americans keep beef on the table. And Americans experimented with legumes, beans, and chicken to add more protein and substance to their meals. Dishes such as spaghetti with meatless marinara or other sauce, once thought of as nutritionally inferior because of the lack of meat, were now being used as alternatives to the typical steak and potatoes dinner.

Beef: The Nutritional Powerhouse?

It's a common perception in American culture that people need to eat beef to meet their bodies' needs for protein and other vital nutrients. We often point to the lore of the Wild West and say, "See! They ate beef all the time and they looked strong and healthy!" But, as discussed, those hardy pioneers didn't really eat that much beef, at least not compared to modern consumption. In fact, Americans ate 75 percent more beef at the end than at the start of the 1900s.

Yes, your body needs protein, vitamins, and minerals to function properly. But do those essential nutrients need to come from beef? No, not all. Let's look at protein. In general, 1 ounce of any kind meat—be it in the form of beef, chicken, pork, fish, turkey, or even an egg (which is about 1 ounce)—contains 7 grams of protein. Beef is no higher in protein than any other kind of meat mentioned. In fact, beef may actually be a *poorer* source of protein when fat content is factored into the picture. If you go beyond generalities and look at different cuts of meat, you'll find that fat becomes a competing element, making less room for protein in that ounce of meat! For example, if you eat 1 ounce of roasted skinless white meat chicken, you've consumed about 8 grams of protein. Eat 1 ounce of roasted prime rib, and you're down to about 6 grams of protein. These differences may not seem like much when you're looking at just 1 ounce, but as those ounces add up so do the differences. By the time you get to a "standard" serving size of 3½ ounces, that prime rib gives you just 21 grams of protein, whereas the skinless chicken breast gives you 28 grams of protein. (See Chapter 5 for more about protein and beef.)

And what about iron? While beef has been famously prescribed as a dietary treatment for, or a preventative means against developing, iron-deficiency anemia, beef is not the *only* good source of iron. (See Chapter 5 for more about iron and beef.) All animal meats—poultry, fish, pork, beef, and egg yolk—are excellent sources of iron, ounce for ounce. In fact, some animal sources, such as clams, contain *higher* amounts of iron per ounce than some beef cuts, such as sirloin steak (3 ounces of steamed clams contains about 24 milligrams of iron; the same amount of sirloin steak contains about 3 milligrams of iron).

Although beef may show slightly higher numbers of iron than some other animal meats such as chicken (1 ounce of prime rib contains about 3 milligrams of iron compared to 1 milligram of iron in the same amount of chicken breast), if you weigh in the issue of calories, the gain in iron content may not be as superior as it seems. That ounce of roasted prime rib contains 80 calories. Yet 1 ounce of roasted skinless chicken breast or 1 ounce of steamed clams contains about 40 calories—half that of the prime rib! Eating the chicken breast will leave more caloric room in your diet to focus on other iron-containing foods, especially those iron-packed plant foods—like whole grains (such as fortified whole-grain cereals), dark leafy vegetables (such as Swiss chard), and dried fruits (such as prunes).

It's true that the iron in beef, poultry, pork, and fish is readily absorbable by the body. But the iron in plant foods is easily made more available when they're eaten along with animal foods (for example, in a bean and chicken dish) or foods high in vitamin C (such as strawberries and oranges). Increasing the proportion of plant foods in your diet is a must, especially if you want to help stave off the common chronic diseases, including heart disease, and many forms of cancers. So it is very beneficial to balance your daily caloric intake to emphasize foods from plant sources.

Many women, especially those who are still menstruating or who are pregnant, need to keep a close eye on their iron intake. Men, however, do not need as much iron as women do. The Recommended Dietary Allowance, or RDA, of iron is 10 milligrams for the average adult male, but it's 15 milligrams for premenopausal women and 30 milligrams for pregnant women.

Consuming too much iron, however, can actually be quite harmful. Some researchers believe that an excess iron intake can lead to heart disease. And there is a serious, common heredity disorder that is not as well known as it should be: hemachromatosis. This disorder impairs the body's ability to metabolize iron effectively. The result is that dangerously high amounts of iron can build up in the blood, potentially leading to serious liver, kidney, and heart damage. So, while iron is indeed important for many women and children, it should not be overly emphasized in the diet of others.

Beef: A Real Man's Meat?

Want big, strong biceps, triceps, quads, abs, and pecs? Eat beef. Lots and lots of beef. So goes common wisdom, disseminated freely in gyms and on athletic fields everywhere. Red meat has longed been considered a *man's* meat, its blood-juices conjuring images of conquest and triumph. Ancient Greeks staged the glory of battle, dressing themselves in skins and horns and attacking the bull that was to become their dinner. They bathed in the blood of the kill and then ate of its flesh, believing that doing so imbued them with the bull's strength and courage. This perception that beef is a manly meat, a source of potency and vigor, persists even in modern times.

Beef for muscle building sounds logical. What's muscle, anyway? Protein. Ah, well, let's eat some steak! Beef is also a source of vitamins (such as vitamin B_{12}) and minerals (such as iron), and those ads for athletic-performance products certainly tell us that we need vitamins and minerals. Give me some more steak, and let's get some muscle tone!

Well, not so fast. The truth is, it's not really what you eat that defines your muscle size and tone. You can't build muscle mass by eating muscle (unless you're building up your gastronomic muscle). You build and shape your muscles only by exercising them. It's what you *do*, not what you eat, that sculpts your physique. Nothing—absolutely nothing—that you eat (or don't eat) will give you a body builder's body. Only months, and often years, of structured physical activity will accomplish such a goal.

Diet comes into the game as a means of providing energy to supply your muscle-gaining activity—but not a diet that is high in protein. In fact, a diet that is excessively high in protein, either through a high beef diet or protein/amino acid supplements, might instead diminish athletic performance and cause health problems. Increasing your consumption of amino acids doesn't build more muscle. Rather, excessive protein in your diet can cause your body to work harder to remove metabolic waste, potentially leading to dehydration.

If you want to bulk up, try carbohydrates—and not necessarily the carbohydrates found in a typical sports drink or sports bar. Just go for the carbohydrates found in whole grains, fruits, legumes, and vegetables. The American Dietetic Association (ADA) recommends for an athlete's diet that 60 to 65 percent of the total caloric intake should be from carbohydrate sources, ideally the carbohydrates found in plant foods. Hard-core athletes should consume up to 70 percent of their daily calories as carbohydrates. Carbohydrates help your muscles maintain their glycogen stores, providing an energy reserve they can draw from on demand for aerobic and anaerobic activities.

You may have heard of the notion of "carbohydrate loading," by which athletes, such as marathon runners, sit down to large pasta dinners the night before a big race. What these athletes are doing is beefing (no pun intended) up their glycogen stores—or, rather, their muscle energy stores—to competitively get them through a long period of muscle activity. Eating a balanced daily diet that emphasizes complex carbohydrates and provides adequate calories can easily keep muscle glycogen stores intact and keep you feeling healthy and energetic for all of your daily activities.

Of course, everyone's individual dietary needs are unique. If you want to increase your athletic performance (or have any kind of special dietary need), seek the advice of a registered dietitian to make sure that what you eat meets your specific requirements. And a balanced diet—one containing adequate servings of fruits, vegetables, and whole grains as well as enough protein (meat or plant sources) to meet your Recommended Dietary Allowances—is the best way for you to give your body the fuel it needs to build strong, healthy muscles and other tissues.

Dressed for Dinner: The Many Ways Beef Comes to the Table

Little wonder we eat so much beef, with all the many ways it's served! The beef industry identifies about 300 different cuts of beef, the names of which often vary among the different regions of the United States. A typical meat counter might offer 30 to 50 different cuts. Although you can make any cut of meat more lean by trimming all visible fat from the edges before cooking it, where on the cow the meat comes from can make a tremendous difference in its fat content. In general, cuts with the names "loin" and "round" are usually leaner than other cuts.

The U.S. Department of Agriculture's (USDA's) voluntary grading system rates beef cuts as Prime, Choice, and Select. For the same cut of beef, a Prime grade has more fat (as much as 40 percent more than a Select grade), which is what gives them their tender texture and rich flavor. This is often visible as marbling—veins of fat that traverse the piece of beef. Choice grade has less fat than Prime grade and 5 to 20 percent more fat than Select grade of the same cut. The cut of beef is an important factor when considering fat content. Here are the most common types of cuts and their general characteristics:

Brisket. The brisket is from the front of the breast and just above the front legs of the cow. This cut is typically high in fat content, coming in at 8 to 10 grams of fat per cooked ounce.

Chuck. The chuck is cut from the cow's shoulder and neck areas.

The fat content ranges from 3 to 8 grams of fat per cooked ounce, depending whether the grade is Select or Choice.

Flank. Flank steak comes from the bottom sides of the cow. It's fairly lean if trimmed to zero visible fat before it's cooked—4 to 7 grams of fat per cooked ounce. London broil steak is a flank cut, and some ground beef is made from flank meat. The cooking process also determines the final leanness of a flank steak. Dry-heat methods of cooking, such as broiling and grilling, produce a relatively lean meal, but cooking in moist heat, such as braising, usually means the meat is coated in its own fatty juices.

Loin. The loin comes from the top side of the cow, near the spine between the hip and the start of the ribs. Loin meat is tasty and tender, and some loin cuts are the most expensive cuts of beef you can buy. There are many different types of loin meat, and they differ in their degree of leanness. Short loin cuts include the tenderloin (otherwise known as filet mignon), which is very lean at about 3 grams of fat per cooked ounce. Other short loin cuts are the top loin, porterhouse, T-bone, and top loin steaks, which all are generally lean if the visible fat is trimmed away before cooking. Sirloin is the other category of loin meats. Examples of sirloin include boneless sirloin, wedge-bone sirloin, and flat-bone sirloin. Again the degree of leanness depends on the amount of fat that is trimmed before cooking or eating. However, sirloin is generally higher in fat than short loin.

Rib. As the name indicates, rib meat is from around the ribs of the cow. This meat is tender but rather high in fat—6 to 10 grams of fat per cooked ounce, depending on the grade and amount of fat around the edges of the cut when cooking. Rib-eye roasts and steaks and rib steaks and roasts are examples of this type of beef.

Round. Round cuts come from the back end of the cow. This meat, such as eye of round, top round, and round steak, is generally lean, ranging from 1 (very low!) to 5 grams of fat per cooked ounce. Other examples of round cuts are boneless rump roast, cubed steak, and ground round.

Shank. The shank is meat from the cow's legs. Shank meat is tough and sinewy but fairly lean at 2 to 4 grams of fat per cooked ounce. Examples of shank meat include shank cross cuts and shank stew meat.

The most often consumed form of beef is ground beef, commonly known as hamburger. Much ground beef comes from chuck and other pieces not suitable for sale or eating in any other form, and often has trimmings and other by-products added to enhance flavor and texture. Regular ground beef is 16 to 20 percent fat; extra-lean ground beef can have as little as 7 percent fat content. The National Restaurant Association reports that the hamburger sandwich is the most popular item in restaurants, appearing on 75 percent of all menus.

Ground beef is particularly vulnerable to food-borne pathogens (more on this in later chapters) and should always be cooked to well done if you choose to eat it. Because of the threat of mad cow disease, more correctly known as bovine spongiform encephalopathy (BSE), many health experts recommend avoiding ground beef products in Europe and other locations where BSE is known to exist (or to avoid it altogether anywhere, anytime).

Other beef products include organ meats and trimmed elements, such as tails, known collectively as offal. Favored organ meats include brains, tongues, eyes, testicles, intestines, stomach linings (tripe), heart, liver, and kidneys. And let's not overlook headcheese, which combines many of these elements into a sort of sausage loaf. Once especially popular in Europe, offal has fallen out of favor as a consequence of concerns over BSE. (See Chapter 2 for more on BSE and other diseases.)

Beef jerky is made of strips of beef, usually from cuts that can't be sold or eaten in any other form, which is dried and sometimes smoked or flavored. Beef jerky is often high in both fat and sodium (salt). In America, it is typically sold as a snack food.

Veal is the meat of a calf slaughtered at around 3 months of age, before its weight goes over 150 pounds (adult cattle, typically slaughtered around 2 years of age, weigh between 1,000 and 1,500 pounds). Veal is pale in color compared to beef and more nutritionally dense. As is the case with beef, the fat content of veal depends on the cut, and how much fat is trimmed before the cooking process. In general, loin and round cuts are the leanest, with 1 to 4 grams of fat per cooked ounce.

Beyond Burgers and Steaks

Eliminating red meat from your diet will not necessarily distance you from beef when it comes to your food supply. Beef by-products show up in an amazing variety of non-meat food items, including gelatins, marshmallows, candy, mayonnaise, chewing gum, yogurt, cookies, and many low-fat or "light" products. And natural sausage casings, though rarely used in modern sausage-making, are made from beef intestines. Even sausage and other meat products that you might not think of as containing beef often do. While some turkey sausage products are 100 percent turkey and use pork casings, for example, others such as turkey kielbasa often contain small to moderate amounts of beef to add texture and flavor. Always check the label, ask the butcher, or contact the manufacturer if you are uncertain about the beef content of *any* sausage product.

Beef and beef products are also key ingredients in the 20 billion or so hot dogs Americans consume each year. The hot dog is actually a kind of sausage made by blending meat and meat by-products (sometimes just beef, most often beef and pork, and sometimes poultry) along with spices and seasonings into a batter-like mixture. The mixture is then pumped into casings (once made from intestines but now typically removable cellophane), cooked, smoked, and cooled. Though variations on the hot dog have been around for more than 500 years (known as the "dachshund sausage"), it wasn't until the 1904 World's Fair in St. Louis, Missouri, that a vendor served these "hot dogs" in long buns, creating the hot dog as we know it today.

Not surprisingly, hot dogs are quite high in fat, with the typical fat content running from 14 to 17 percent. In recent years, hot-dog manufacturers have come out with reduced-fat, low-fat (1 to 7 percent fat), and even no-fat hot dogs in an effort to appeal to today's health-conscious consumers. The industry sells 41 million pounds of these lower-fat and no-fat hot dogs a year, which accounts for about 15 percent of overall hot-dog sales.

Hot dogs made in the United States typically contain ingredients banned in hot dogs made in Europe, sometimes including mechanically extracted meat, which can be contaminated with spinal cord tissue as well as by-products. Because scientists believe spinal cord tissue is one of the most concentrated locations for the infectious agent that causes BSE, European regulations prohibit using mechanical extraction to prevent such contamination. Some health officials recommend avoiding hot dogs containing any beef products as the safest preventive measure. If you are unsure about the beef content of a hot-dog product, once again, check the label, ask your butcher, or contact the manufacturer.

Changing Lifestyles, Changing Tastes

Through much of the twentieth century, Americans looked on their eating habits as indicators of health and prosperity. This came in good part from a long history of similar perspectives in other Western cultures, particularly Europe. Voluptuousness—big bodies—was much desired and admired well into the 1950s before trends shifted to favor thinner physiques. Some of the change came about as a result of new discoveries in physiology and medicine. As scientists and doctors gained a more sophisticated understanding of how the human body functions in health and in sickness, they began to realize that centuries of fashionable obesity had done little to extend the length of quality of human life. In fact, it had done the opposite.

These discoveries came as consumption of beef—as well as of sugar and processed foods—was on the increase. Beef consumption peaked at an average of 72 pounds per person in 1980; since then, it has fallen off to around 63 pounds. Most researchers attribute the decline in eating beef (and other red meat) to heightened awareness of the health consequences of a diet high in red meat (especially of the higher-fat varieties), including increased risk of heart disease, stroke, and cancer.

As beef consumption declined, the beef industry countered with changes and improvements of its own. New herd-management techniques, coupled with newly developed breeds of cattle, have resulted in cows that are both larger and leaner than their predecessors. In 2000, cows were as much as 27 percent leaner than the cows of 1980, according to industry sources. Some new breeds of cattle provide beef cuts with half the calories and a fourth the fats of beef from before. And today's cattle are more efficient in terms of edible product. In 2000, a cow produced considerably more beef than did a cow in 1975.

Declining beef consumption has also caused the beef industry to look for ways to reclaim market share. In addition to feeding and breeding changes, efforts meeting with success include the following:

Convenience foods. Prepackaged, ready-to-fix beef entrées are now sold fresh from the grocery store cold cases. This strategy capitalizes on the increasing number of women in the workforce. Families' frequent complaints about "What's for dinner?" are often among the day's most challenging questions.

Advertising. Aggressive promotional campaigns have been developed to spread the word about the new leaner beef. This strategy highlights the nutritional benefits of eating beef within the nutritional guidelines established by the USDA, the federal Health and Human Services Division, the American Heart Association, and other agencies.

Nutrition. The industry has focused on specific nutritional targets, such as iron deficiency among women of childbearing age. This strategy emphasizes the high iron content of beef and encourages women to make beef products part of a balanced, nutritious diet.

Breeding. Breeders have developed new hybrids, such as the beefalo, a cross between a buffalo and a cow. Beefalo meat is higher in protein and lower in saturated fats than conventional beef. It's a tough sell to consumers, however, who are accustomed to beef that looks and tastes like the beef they've grown to enjoy.

Beef around the World

Eating beef as a regular part of the daily diet has always been primarily a Western habit. Eastern cultures, such as traditional Japanese and Chinese populations, have generally been more inclined toward a diet with a high plant-based content, though also including fish and some poultry. U.S. beef and veal exports increased eightfold between 1980 and 1990, with significant penetration into markets in Asia. Some researchers worry that this globalization of beef consumption will (and already has begun to) disturb nutritional balances as well as ecosystems. Cattle eat significant quantities of corn and other grains and graze on millions of acres of grasslands around the world. What affect does this have on human populations? Researchers are still studying this question; no one as yet knows the answer.

Along with the globalization of beef consumption has been the globalization of diseases that were once limited to countries such as the United States, where people eat a large amount of animal protein (mostly in the form of beef) and relatively little whole-plant foods. Health experts worry about the effect the increased beef consumption will have on people who have traditionally not had beef as a part of their daily diet. There have already been detectable rises in the rates for stomach cancer, which is thought to be linked to dietary changes including increased beef consumption, in countries such as Japan. (See Chapter 4 for more on beef and your health.) Heart disease and many forms of cancers are on the increase in places such as Asia and the Mediterranean region, where they had previously been uncommon. Indeed, it seems that in locations where people deviate from their traditional ways of eating, including eating more beef and less plant-based foods, the rates for these diseases have been rising.

Environmental Issues

In addition to the growing health concerns of increased beef consumption around the world, there are also environmental concerns. Critics of the worldwide cattle industry say large-scale cattle farming has destroyed millions of acres of otherwise productive land through grazing. Scientists have raised concerns about water contamination from sewage runoff. And animal activists charge that slaughtering practices common in the United States are cruel and inhumane. These issues remain unresolved.

Consumer groups have expressed much concern through the years about the use of hormones, antibiotics, vaccines, and other substances that intend to make the lives of cattle and other livestock raised for food healthier and more productive. (At present, cattle manufacturers in the United States can use certain hormones in limited doses to encourage growth but can use antibiotics only to treat illness and must certify that an animal has been antibiotic-free for a specified period before slaughter.) The gains have been significant and impressive. A steer raised for beef in 1975 yielded 475 pounds of meat, whereas a steer raised in 1999 yielded over 600 pounds of meat—a quite hefty increase. Analysts attribute this increase to improved animal husbandry, from breeding programs that produce larger animals to control over the animal's environment from birth to slaughter to changes in animal nutrition and feed. Critics question whether these practices have contributed to the emergence of new and deadly pathogens; scientists are as yet unable to provide definitive answers.

Making Healthy, Educated Choices

Beef alternatives are gaining in popularity. Poultry consumption has increased threefold since the 1950s and continues to climb. Vegan (vegetable-based) meat substitutes have enjoyed dramatic improvements in texture and flavor since they first debuted in the American marketplace in the early 1960s. Soy substitutes can taste, smell, and feel almost like the "real" thing, especially when cooked in dishes with other foods, such as vegetables. Restaurants in cities around the United States, such as Seattle, San Francisco, Boston, Chicago, New York, and Washington, D.C., feature meat-free cuisine that is as good to eat as it is good for you.

The goal of making educated choices about what you eat and don't eat is not to put the beef industry out of business. Rather, the goal is to create a nutritious balance in your daily diet that will support a long and healthy life. Knowledge is power, and gaining more knowledge about how what goes past your lips affects the rest of your body is empowering. After all, it's your body and your life, and you should be able to take care of both as you desire.

2

Is Beef Safe?

During the twentieth century, beef became big business in the United States. So big, in fact, that by the start of the twenty-first century, the American cattle industry produced 26.8 billion pounds of beef and beef products—25 percent of the world's beef supply. Americans spent more than $52 million to buy beef in 2000, an amount that averaged out to nearly $200 per person—the highest level of spending for beef in America's history. To function at this level, cattle operations have become manufacturing centers, not farms. Raising cattle is a specialized production operation that conveys the animals through each step from breeding to slaughter.

Butchering one cow at a time is a fairly straightforward process, as was generally the practice on the small and family farms that made up most of the cattle industry at the opening of the twentieth century. As often as not, he who wielded the knife of slaughter had also been present at the animal's first breath. This farmer knew everything about the cow—its eating habits, living conditions, weight, and illnesses. Cattle grazed the farmer's fields and ate grain the farmer raised. Sometimes meat was bad and made people sick, of course, though this was more likely the result of inadequate preservation (meat not kept cold enough during storage and shipping) than of bacteria from poor sanitation practices during slaughter and dressing (preparing the meat into cuts). As well, herds were relatively small—a few dozen to a few hundred head for the majority of farms. Cows had reasonable room to roam, and nature could manage the waste they produced.

Slaughtering and processing hundreds of cattle an hour—thousands in a day—is an assembly-line production that requires precision and timing. There is little room for challenges such as animals that resist or aren't adequately stunned before slaughter. In the press to move through this volume of cattle, it's frighteningly easy for slips and miscues to occur. Numerous investigations—by news agencies, groups concerned about animal welfare issues, and health officials—have exposed the dark side of America's beef industry. The cattle industry and government agencies are working to eliminate health risks and other problems. These efforts have met with mixed success, and both sides agree that room remains for improvement.

While much of the nation's food supply reaches consumers pathogen free and safe to eat, the U.S. Centers for Disease Control and Prevention (CDC) reports that each year food-borne infections are known to cause 78 million Americans to become ill and more than 5,000 to die. This number may not be a true representation of the actual number of cases, as many of the symptoms of food-borne illness resemble those of the flu. It's unfortunately common to become sick from the food you've eaten without knowing the true cause of your illness. And because most people recover from such bouts quickly and completely, they don't see doctors to confirm what's ailing them. Health experts estimate that there might well be as many as five times more cases of food-borne illnesses than are diagnosed and reported.

More than 250 pathogens—bacteria, viruses, parasites, and other agents that cause disease—can cause food-borne illnesses with various degrees of symptoms, and new sources of infection emerge each year. Many of the pathogens that cause food-borne illnesses today were unknown before the 1970s. Scientists speculate that their appearance has much to do with changes in the beef industry to improve efficiency. Though the diseases that challenge our society are relatively recent, food-borne illness is not a modern phenomenon. When America entered the twentieth century, marveling at the potential of the new industrial economy, diseases such as typhoid fever and botulism were common—and often deadly. Diarrhea and enteritis (inflammation of the intestinal tract), often attributable to "bad" food or water, made up the third leading cause of death in 1900. Refrigeration amounted to placing food on blocks of ice in the summer or outdoors in the winter, resulting in inconsistent temperatures that often ended up at levels that supported, rather than discouraged, bacterial growth. Discoveries such as pasteurization and chlorination improved conditions significantly, as did the advent of indoor refrigerators with freezer compartments (which debuted in the 1920s). These advancements virtually eradicated some of these common diseases.

But while we've conquered the killers of the twentieth century, we must now contend with the killers of the twenty-first century. Most of the pathogens that afflict our modern society are agents that first appeared since about 1980: *Escherichia coli* O157:H7, *Listeria monocytogenes, Campylobacter,* and new variants of *Salmonella.* Most healthy people recover from food-borne illnesses without long-term problems. People who have a high risk for becoming ill after exposure to food-borne pathogens or experiencing complications after illness include the following groups:

- Children under age 4, because their immune systems aren't fully developed yet.
- Elderly adults, because their immune systems are less effective or because they might have chronic or recurring health problems.
- Anyone with a serious or chronic health condition, such as cancer, whose immune system is occupied with fighting the challenge of a potentially life-threatening disease.
- Anyone with an immune system disorder (such as lupus or HIV/AIDS) or who is taking immunosuppressive drugs (such as after an organ transplant).

Most localities (cities, counties, or states) have mandatory reporting requirements for specified food-borne illnesses such as *E. coli* infections, listeriosis, and salmonellosis. This helps public health officials track outbreaks of these illnesses to better understand how they occur and to work to prevent them in the general population. It also provides a way for health-care providers to share information about an infection's typical course and about treatments, either successful or unsuccessful. The CDC gathers and reports data about food-borne illnesses as well as myriad other conditions that reflect the overall health status of Americans.

How Food-Borne Illnesses Happen

While ravaging diseases such as mad cow disease and *E. coli* grab headlines and strike fear in the hearts of beef-eaters nationwide, it's more ordinary and less dramatic illnesses, such as salmonellosis and listeriosis, that sicken (and sometimes kill) more people. Consumers can prevent many food-borne illnesses through proper handling and preparation. Cooking beef thoroughly and to an adequately high temperature (to an internal temperature of around 160°F) kills most bacteria—a practice not especially popular in a culture that loves its steaks and burgers rare.

Often the chain of contamination begins somewhere in the manufacturing process. With hundreds of cows an hour moving through slaughter, intestinal contents and fecal material can splatter onto the meat. Although washing procedures in beef-manufacturing plants clean much of this kind of contamination and random laboratory testing catches some, tainted beef does occasionally slip through and ends up packaged in the grocery store. When laboratory results detect pathogens in tested beef, the manufacturer and the U.S. Department of Agriculture (USDA) issue a recall alert. This requires stores to return the identified lots to the manufacturer. In many instances (though certainly not all), manufacturers are able to intercept the tainted lots at the wholesaler, before they even reach consumers.

Modern production, storage, and transportation methods mean beef can travel vast distances in a short time. Hamburger ground and packed in a plant in Kansas today can be at regional wholesalers serving retail locations in multiple states within 48 hours and distributed to grocery stores the following day. By the time laboratory tests detect the presence of pathogens, the tainted beef is often well on its way to market. A particular problem with ground beef is that modern manufacturing processes generate batches of hamburger that contain meat from potentially thousands of cows. If just one carcass among them is contaminated, the pathogens will taint the entire lot—which could be distributed to numerous wholesalers and retailers before being discovered. Any of these factors, and particularly several of them in combination, can make it difficult for health officials to identify an outbreak when it occurs—victims can be in several states and become ill over a period of several weeks or longer.

Most contaminated meat doesn't look, smell, or taste (after cooking) spoiled. And proper cooking kills most pathogens, so even if you eat beef from a lot later named in a recall, the odds are good that you won't get sick as long as you cooked the meat thoroughly (especially ground beef). It's a good practice, however, to check any beef you have in your refrigerator or freezer every time there is a recall. If you find items that match the recalled lot or batch numbers, return them to the store where you purchased them. The store will either offer you a replacement or refund your money.

The best way to avoid food-borne illness is to be sure the foods you eat are free from contamination—and to eat foods for which the risk of contamination is low. You're reading this book because you want to reduce or eliminate the amount of beef in your diet. An added benefit of doing this is that you will also decrease your chances for developing illnesses—mild or life threatening—that beef-borne pathogens can cause.

Beef Itself Is Not "Bad"

Beef is not inherently bad or bad for you, of course. Beef contains many nutrients that the human body can use; and it can be part of a nutritious diet, as best we understand our bodies' needs, as long as you use lean cuts and keep your portions small. The truth is, however, that we really don't know the long-term health effects of eating the beef that's grown and produced in our modern society. The steak that sizzles on your grill is nothing like the beef that came to the table 100—or even 20—years ago. The interrelationship among diet, nutrition, and health is complex and one that we have only fairly recently begun to untangle.

We will discuss beef consumption and chronic health diseases, such as heart disease and cancer, in later chapters. This chapter focuses on the risks of food-borne infection from eating beef. These risks carry different degrees of likelihood of occurrence as well as potential for severity of illness. This is because our topic is *beef*. Other foods besides beef, particularly those of animal origin, can and do carry food-borne pathogens. Other meats as well as fruits, vegetables, and even water have the potential to cause illness and death. The overwhelming majority of beef products available commercially in the United States, from cuts of beef to hamburger to lunch meats, are safe to eat (from a food-borne illness perspective) as long as you handle and cook them properly. But it is important that you know what risks come with eating beef and how to reduce the likelihood that any of them will cause you and your family members to become ill.

Safeguarding America's Beef Supply

In 1906, Upton Sinclair's novel *The Jungle* gave the world an inside look at the inhumane and unhealthy conditions in Chicago's slaughterhouses at the start of the twentieth century. The fictional tale of an immigrant slaughterhouse worker was vivid and grim, and it horrified the public. One outcome of the public scrutiny that followed the book's publication was the Meat Inspection Act, passed in 1906, which required federal inspection of slaughterhouses and beef products. (Also passed in 1906 was the Pure Food and Drug Act, which prohibited actions to adulterate food and mislabel it.) The USDA became the enforcement agency for the resulting guidelines and procedures, which cover nearly every aspect of beef production from breeding to slaughter.

The procedures these two pieces of federal legislation established stayed in place for nearly a century, until once again public outcry forced more change. The 1990s saw a number of severe outbreaks of *E. coli* infections that sickened hundreds of people in numerous states and resulted in a dozen or so deaths. Investigators traced the infections, several of which involved hamburgers served at fast-food chain restaurants, to meat contaminated in the manufacturing process.

At the time of the *E. coli* outbreaks, the meat safety inspection system that was in place had USDA inspectors working in nearly every beef-manufacturing plant in the United States. It was their responsibility to oversee the slaughter and packaging processes, inspect carcasses and beef cuts for obvious contamination, and conduct sporadic testing for microbes such as *E. coli* and *Salmonella*. But it was a system that relied on the "poke and sniff" approach, as industry watchers dubbed the standard method. Even though research and technological advances had turned up new, more sophisticated methods for testing meat to detect unseen bacterial contamination, beef manufacturers were reluctant to incorporate them (though some did so on a limited basis). The new tests cost money and didn't help the manufacturer comply with federal regulations. And USDA inspectors couldn't require manufacturers to use the new tests because the law didn't give them the authority to do so.

After the high-profile outbreaks of meat-borne infections of the 1990s, public attention once again targeted the beef-manufacturing industry. The USDA decided to shift inspection and monitoring efforts to a preventive model called Hazard Analysis and Critical Control Point (HACCP). With HACCP, the USDA felt it established a kind of partnership with beef manufacturers and began holding the industry more directly accountable for monitoring their own compliance with regulations and safe slaughter practices. This new approach shifted emphasis to monitoring key points within the beef production process. Under HACCP, federal inspectors focus on potential major health and safety problems, while manufacturers conduct routine pathogen testing. Compliance has become a blend of honor and enforcement. Supporters say HACCP works better than the old system because it holds beef manufacturers directly accountable for conditions within their plants, but critics contend HACCP is akin to putting a dog on duty to guard a henhouse.

While there have been improvements in beef safety in recent years, problems remain. Critics charge—and even the USDA acknowledges—that the current system lacks the resources and sometimes the authority to take the drastic measures it would require to bring pathogen contamination to near-zero levels. Meat recalls are on the rise, with each year setting a new record. Some of this increase is no doubt the result of improved and more sensitive laboratory tests as well as the shift to HACCP, although the situation continues to concern public health officials. News stories contain report after report about beef-manufacturing plants that are frequent offenders, repeatedly violating pathogen levels and safe handling procedures. In nearly every meat-borne illness outbreak that has occurred in recent years, investigators have uncovered a pattern of problems and violations at the manufacturer.

In one 2000 case, for example, USDA inspectors issued hundreds of citations to a plant for incidents of fecal contamination and other violations over the course of 10 months and even suspended the plant's operations on several occasions. Yet, in the end, 500 people became ill, more than 20 were hospitalized, and 1 child died—the consequence of beef contaminated with *E. coli* that was shipped to a restaurant that then failed to follow safe handling procedures.

But the shortcomings aren't only on the production side. This scenario illustrates yet another dimension of the complex problem: preparation. Even if the beef that leaves the manufacturer is contaminated, it has only the *potential* to cause illness, because cooking at an appropriately high temperature (above 160°F) kills nearly all of the pathogens. Had the aforementioned restaurant followed safe handling procedures, no one would have gotten sick—and in fact, we might not have even known that there had been a contamination. But the restaurant's employees used the same knives and cutting boards to cut fruit that they had just used to cut meat—with dire consequences. (Later in this

chapter, see "How Safe Is Your Kitchen?" for more about safe beef handling and preparation procedures.)

In 1997 the Food and Drug Administration (FDA) approved, and
in 1999 the USDA authorized, irradiation as a means to reduce
pathogen contamination (bacteria and parasites) in beef products,
including sausage and lunch meats. Irradiation exposes beef to a high-
frequency electromagnetic radiation called gamma radiation. Gamma-
rays belong to the same family of energy waves as visible light and
radio frequencies. At the doses approved for irradiation, which are very
low, gamma radiation does not leave residual radioactivity behind. A
simplistic view of irradiation is that it selectively "cooks" bacteria such
as E. coli, Salmonella, and Listeria without altering other cellular structures in the meat—much as a microwave oven can thaw frozen foods
without cooking them. All irradiated food products must carry prominent labeling identifying them as such.

While organizations such as the American Medical Association and
the American Dietetic Association support food irradiation, the
method has many critics. Some consumer groups are concerned that a
process that focuses on killing pathogens after they already contami-
nate beef shifts attention away from issues of sanitation in the manufacturing process. They believe a more effective approach is to target
the causes of contamination by improving conditions and practices in
slaughterhouses and packing plants. Other groups and individuals have
negative associations with the concept of radiation, viewing it as something that causes cancer or mass destruction. And some people resist
the idea of doing anything to food that is unnatural—that is, presents
food items in forms not occurring in nature.

Yet in more than 40 years of research and testing that lies behind
food irradiation practices, scientists have not been able to identify any
adverse consequences of irradiation. There is less nutrient loss than
occurs with pasteurization. Irradiation does cause very minor, cell-level
changes in foods. But, in a 1993 report from the American Medical
Association, irradiated food was considered to be "safe and nutritionally adequate" because "the process of irradiation will not introduce

changes in the composition of the food which . . . would impose an adverse effect on human health . . . and will not introduce nutrient losses in the composition of the food, which, from a nutritional point of view, would impose an adverse effect on the nutritional status of individuals or populations." In fact, any chemical change is so inconsequential that scientists have as yet been unable to develop a test to determine whether a food item has been irradiated. Health officials believe that eventually irradiation will parallel pasteurization in terms of positive effects on public health and the food supply.

When Beef Makes You Sick

Beef can make you sick. Thousands of pathogens love to call beef home; and they can cause problems for you, ranging from mild intestinal upset to serious infections. While you can prevent many beef-borne illnesses through proper handling and preparation, infections such as salmonellosis, listeriosis, and *E. coli* remain significant public health problems in the United States and around the world. Rare new diseases, such as bovine spongiform encephalopathy (BSE)—more familiarly known as mad cow disease—are surfacing as well. We won't fully understand the risks and consequences of some food-borne infections for quite some time, until research provides us with more answers and time provides us with more experience in diagnosing, treating, and especially preventing such illnesses. This chapter discusses the most common beef-borne infections—salmonellosis, listeriosis, campylobacteriosis, and *E. coli*—as well as two diseases that receive much press—BSE, which causes the very rare variant Creutzfeldt-Jakob disease (vCJD), and foot and mouth disease, which devastates livestock herds but doesn't infect people (as far as scientists know).

It's not our intent to scare you away from beef by filling a chapter (and your head) with horror stories. Instead, we want to inform you about beef's risks, including the risk of contracting diseases, so you can make educated decisions—based in fact—about what role you want beef to have in your diet. The risk for beef-borne infection is just one facet of eating beef that you must consider. Knowledge about beef-borne illness and about other risks that we discuss in later chapters arms you to make choices about the risks you are willing to confront.

BEEF-BORNE ILLNESSES

Infection	Cases per Year (United States)	Symptoms and Onset	Duration and Outcome
Salmonellosis	2 million, possibly as as many as 4 million	Severe headache, vomiting, intestinal cramps, diarrhea, and fever that begins 6–72 hours after exposure	Most people recover within 7 days; however, about 2,000 deaths result each year.
Listeriosis	2,500 cases of serious illness; unknown number of mild cases	Fever, chills, headache, and backache that begin 1 day to several weeks after exposure	Most people recover within 7–10 days; however, risk of serious complications is high and about 500 deaths result each year.
Campylobacteriosis	2 million, possibly as many as 4 million	Vomiting, intestinal cramps, and diarrhea that begin 2–5 days after exposure	Most people recover within 1 week; however about 500 deaths result each year.
E. coli 0157:H7 infection	73,000	Severe abdominal cramps and bloody diarrhea that begin 3–9 days after exposure	Approximately 95 percent recover within 2 weeks, 5 percent develop serious complications and about 600 who do die each year.
Variant Creutzfeldt-Jakob disease, caused by BSE	More than 100 known cases in the world documented since 1994; none in the United States	Sudden significant emotional or psychiatric problems, weakness, and lack of coordination; unique electroencephalogram disturbances begin 7–10 years after exposure and about 1 year before death	Always fatal.
Foot and mouth disease	Not known to affect humans	Not known to affect humans	Not known to affect humans, though devastating to cloven-hoof livestock.

SALMONELLOSIS

Though precise figures are impossible to calculate because many people who become ill don't go to the doctor or hospital unless their symptoms become severe, about 2 million people are affected by salmonellosis each year and about 2,000 of them die. There are about 2,000 different strains of *Salmonella*, which are all capable of infecting humans. The key symptoms of salmonellosis are severe headache, followed by vomiting, intestinal cramping, diarrhea, and fever. These symptoms can appear from 6 to 72 hours after eating an infected food, and can last for two to seven days. (The bacteria that cause this illness, *Salmonella*, have nothing to do with salmon but rather are named after the American scientist Daniel E. Salmon.)

When it comes to infection, a little bit goes a long way for *Salmonella*. Laboratory studies suggest as few as 15 to 20 organisms are all it takes to cause illness in otherwise healthy people. Most people recover without complications; though in people with weakened immune systems, salmonellosis can be fatal. People with HIV/AIDS are especially susceptible to *Salmonella* infections. A small percentage of those who get salmonellosis go on to develop a condition called Reiter syndrome, in which the joints become inflamed and painful. Reiter syndrome can then develop into a condition called chronic reactive arthritis.

The only treatment for salmonellosis is supportive—being sure to drink enough liquids to replace fluids lost through diarrhea. Severe diarrhea might require hospitalization for treatment with intravenous fluids. Antibiotics aren't usually helpful unless the infection spreads to involve other organs, which is uncommon. In fact, health experts believe the once-common practice of giving cattle antibiotics to prevent illness and promote growth has made possible strains of *Salmonella* that are resistant to antibiotics.

Cooking steaks and roasts to at least a temperature of 145°F (and holding that temperature for 10 minutes, or cooking at higher temperatures if the time of cooking is shorter) and ground beef to 160°F throughout will kill *Salmonella* that beef might harbor. After cooking, be sure not to let steaks, roasts, or ground beef sit at room temperature for too long. If you are not going to eat the meat right away, hold at a temperature that is above 140°F. And thorough hand washing with warm water and soap kills bacteria that get on your skin. While cold temperatures (refrigeration and freezing) prevent *Salmonella* from multiplying, they don't kill the bacteria. People get salmonellosis primarily through *Salmonella*-contaminated beef, chicken, eggs, and unpasteurized milk—a consequence of fecal contamination.

The CDC estimates that salmonellosis costs the United States more than $1 billion a year in direct (medical care) and indirect (lost wages and productivity) expenses. This represents a decline since 1998 when the USDA implemented its HACCP inspection model to target this pathogen. Before 1998 about 7 percent of tested beef turned out positive for *Salmonella* contamination; by 2001 the USDA reported positive results in just half that amount, 3.7 percent. The USDA and the beef industry are hopeful that continued diligence and monitoring will eventually eliminate these organisms from the nation's beef supply.

LISTERIOSIS

Listeria monocytogenes is among the most common contaminants in the human environment. This organism can exist in uncooked meats, in water, in prepared foods such as hot dogs and lunch meats, and even in the soil. Listeriosis, the infection that results from *Listeria* contamination, has potentially serious consequences for pregnant women (in whom it can cause miscarriages and stillbirths) and newborn infants (who can get it from their infected mothers). One-third of diagnosed listeriosis cases are in pregnant women. This infection can also cause serious complications such as meningitis (inflammation of the tissues around the brain) and septicemia (blood poisoning). While *Listeria* contamination exists in beef cuts and beef products such as hamburger, most outbreaks of listeriosis occur from eating products that might be eaten cold or uncooked, such as hot dogs and lunch meats (as well as unpasteurized soft cheeses). Refrigeration slows, but doesn't stop, *Listeria* growth; fortunately, cooking kills the organism. (Cook poultry to 180°F, and fish and other meats to 160°F. Again, hold at a temperature of 140°F if you are not going to eat the meat items right away.)

A 1998 listeriosis outbreak resulted in 15 deaths and 80 hospitalizations, as well as the recall of 35 million pounds of hot dogs and lunch meats, which were determined to be the cause. In 1999, there were more than 30 product recalls for *Listeria* contamination, nearly all involving ready-to-eat meat products. And in 2000, in an effort to reduce the threat of listeriosis, the USDA approved increasing the amounts of three food additives—sodium diacetate, sodium lactate, and potassium lactate—in these prepared meat products to create a more hostile environment for the *Listeria* organism. (But note that if you have high blood pressure or are salt sensitive, you should eliminate foods that contain high amounts of sodium additives. And for general health for everyone, we recommend that less is always better as far as additives go.)

It can take several days to as long as several weeks after eating contaminated food for listeriosis to develop. Symptoms include sudden fever, chills, headache, and backache. Some people also experience abdominal cramping and diarrhea. About 2,500 Americans become seriously ill with listeriosis each year, and 500 of them die. This relatively high fatality rate is one reason listeriosis is so dangerous despite its relatively low infection rate. In addition to pregnant women and newborns, people for whom listeriosis is a serious health threat include those who have cancer, diabetes, kidney disease, and immune system disorders. People with HIV/AIDS are significantly more susceptible than other people to listeriosis and are more likely to develop complications. If you are at high risk for listeriosis (particularly if you are pregnant), avoid eating cold cuts and cold lunch meats (including at restaurants and delis).

What if you eat something that later is recalled for *Listeria* contamination? The odds are good that if you are otherwise healthy, you won't get sick. The CDC says the risk of listeriosis is very slight unless you belong to a high-risk group, in which case you should contact your doctor. A blood test can show whether you have the infection. Doctors usually treat high-risk people with antibiotics, though someone who is otherwise healthy is likely to recover without treatment.

CAMPYLOBACTERIOSIS

While *Campylobacter* infections are the most common cause of bacterial diarrhea in the United States, cases generally occur at random rather than in large outbreaks. To avoid possible contamination, be sure to cook meats to at least 160°F. Also, be sure to drink only pasteurized milk or juice and treated water (public water systems in the United States are treated).

The CDC estimates that there are 2 million cases of campylobacteriosis each year, affecting about 1 percent of the American population. Symptoms of infection include vomiting, abdominal cramping, and diarrhea (sometimes bloody) and usually begin two to five days after exposure. Illness lasts about a week, after which the vast majority of people recover without further complications. As is the case for most infections, people with weakened immune systems are at greater risk for health problems than people who are otherwise healthy. Antibiotics are seldom effective (they must be given early in the course of the disease to have any effect). Chicken is more likely to be the source of campylobacteriosis than beef, although any animal product can carry *Campylobacter* organisms.

The USDA reports that, under its HACCP model, campylobacteriosis is on the decline. Cases decreased 15 percent between 1996, when the agency implemented HACCP, and 1998, the latest year for which data are available.

E. COLI INFECTION

E. coli O157:H7 infections dropped onto the CDC infectious disease radar screen in 1993 with an outbreak in the western United States traced to tainted hamburger products at a fast-food chain restaurant. Four children died and hundreds of other people became ill in the outbreak, which ultimately was traced to unsanitary practices and conditions in a beef-manufacturing plant. The situation focused the eyes of the world on meat handling methods in the United States, resulting in manufacturing changes as well as a massive public education campaign. *E. coli* and other coliform pathogens live in the intestinal tracts of animals and humans. Within this confined environment, they are harmless. But when they spill into other environments, as often happens during the slaughter process, they become dangerous agents of illness.

The CDC reports that each year, more than 73,000 people become ill with *E. coli* infections and 600 of them die as a result. Most people who contract an *E. coli* infection are sick for 5 to 10 days and then fully recover. The primary symptoms are severe abdominal cramping and bloody diarrhea. Those who are very young and those who are very old are at particular risk for a very serious and potentially fatal complication called hemolytic uremic syndrome in which the infection destroys the body's red blood cells and the kidneys fail. About 5 percent of *E. coli* infections lead to this syndrome, which requires intensive medical care, including blood transfusions and kidney dialysis. About 95 percent of the people who get hemolytic uremic syndrome eventually recover, though some have residual medical problems.

Because *E. coli* infections are a public health risk, most localities require doctors to report confirmed and suspected cases. Stool tests confirm the presence of the *E. coli* bacteria, though not all laboratories are equipped to conduct the tests. It is also possible to spread the infection through contact with the feces of infected people, though proper hand washing can negate this risk. Beef is not the only source of *E. coli*. Contamination can occur in other food products as well, most notably unpasteurized fruit juices and in water. Investigators traced several outbreaks of *E. coli* infection in the 1990s to unpasteurized apple cider and sewage-contaminated water.

The risk of illness from *E. coli* contamination is highest for ground beef because the process of making ground beef mixes the meat all together. This spreads the pathogens throughout the meat instead of confining them to the meat's surface. Unless the ground beef is then cooked to an internal temperature of at least 160°F, the likelihood of illness is high. It doesn't take many *E. coli* organisms to cause infection. In beef cuts such as steaks or roasts, however, any *E. coli* generally stay on the surface of the meat where they quickly die when the beef is cooked.

Undercooking and cross-contamination are the most common ways *E. coli* infections spread in people. Burgers cooked to medium well, medium rare, and especially rare do not get hot enough to kill bacteria and can become a source of infection. Contrary to popular belief, beef's color after cooking provides no proof that the cooking temperature was high enough to kill *E. coli* and other bacteria—unless that color is pink, which is proof positive that the meat's internal temperature did not reach 160°F. The only way to know whether the beef reached an adequate temperature is to use a meat thermometer—and while most restaurants do, many home cooks do not.

Cross-contamination during preparation is also a serious risk. In a 2000 outbreak of *E. coli* infection in the Upper Midwest, in which one child died and dozens of people became ill, investigators traced the source to a knife and cutting surface used first for preparing *E. coli*–infected steaks and then for preparing fruit for the restaurant's salad bar. The child who died ate no beef, only the fruit. It is crucial to wash your hands, all utensils, and all cutting surfaces with hot, soapy water before and after use and especially between food items. The best way to prevent cross-contamination is to use one set of utensils and cutting surfaces for beef (and other meats) and another one for other food items, virtually eliminating the possibility of cross-contamination (as long as you thoroughly wash your hands after working with each type of food).

MAD COW DISEASE: BOVINE SPONGIFORM ENCEPHALOPATHY

A 2001 public opinion poll found that 20 percent of Americans had reduced the amount of beef they eat as a direct result of their concerns about BSE, commonly known as mad cow disease—despite the fact that no case has as yet been detected in cattle in the United States. Furthermore, three out of four survey participants said they would give up beef entirely if BSE was discovered in the United States—far more people than those who are willing to give up (or even cut back on) beef because of more common risks that have known and potentially serious health consequences, such as heart disease or even cancer! Why does such an extraordinarily rare disease in cattle frighten people to the point of willing disengagement from a favorite food? Because BSE appears linked to an extraordinarily rare but horrifying disease that does afflict people: variant Creutzfeldt-Jakob disease, the human counterpart to mad cow disease.

BSE attacks the nervous system of a cow, leaving the brain riddled with spongelike holes and pockets. The word *spongiform* means "spongelike." In its early stages, BSE affects brain functions that control behavior, causing infected cows to stumble around and act frightened or aggressive. As it destroys more brain tissue, BSE affects physical movement as well. Eventually, an infected animal becomes aggressive and loses balance and coordination. This is where the name "mad cow" disease comes from—infected animals act "crazy" as the disease progresses. Most often, infected animals are euthanized well before the later stages of the disease, both to provide a humane end to the animal's suffering and to prevent infection of other animals. Without euthanasia, an animal with BSE generally dies within a year after it begins to show symptoms (though it could have had the disease for as long as eight years before showing symptoms).

British veterinarians diagnosed the first case of BSE in a cow in Britain in 1986 and diagnosed about 200,000 animal cases by the time they determined the disease was under control in 1996. Scientists aren't sure how BSE came into existence, but many believe it is a mutation that occurred through contact with a related infectious agent in another species. One theory holds responsible an antelope imported from an African wildlife park. Another theory points the finger at the practice of using slaughter waste as ingredients in animal feed products: In this way bovine feed included by-products from slaughtered sheep that had a brain-wasting disease called scrapie. And some researchers believe that BSE started as a mutation in a single cow, which was spread when that cow's remains were used as ingredient in feed. Nearly all scientists agree, however, that using meat- and bone-meal-enhanced feed made with contaminated by-products is the means by which BSE has spread, and Britain banned the practice of using such feed for cattle in 1988 and for all livestock in 1996.

Although researchers have been able to isolate the agent that causes BSE, they are not certain how to classify it. It is smaller than a conventional virus, yet seems to behave as a protein. Scientists have dubbed this agent a "prion"—a cellular structure that lacks a nucleus and thus carries no genetic material. There is no way to kill infectious prions if they exist in a cow slaughtered for beef. Prions can survive freezing, heat (even temperatures high enough for sterilization), and exposure to antiseptic chemicals—the most common methods for destroying pathogens. This resistance to conventional methods of destruction puzzles both researchers and health officials.

People don't actually get BSE; only cows contract this form of the disease. But people do get other prion-caused diseases, known as transmittable spongiform encephalopathies (TSEs), that produce progressive, degenerative neurological damage ultimately resulting in death. In addition to vCJD, these conditions include classic Creutzfeldt-Jakob disease (CJD); kuru, afflicting an isolated New Guinea population that once engaged in ritual mortuary cannibalism (the eating of human flesh and internal organs after death); Gerstmann-Straussler syndrome, a rare inherited disease caused by a genetic mutation; fatal familial insomnia, a rare inherited disease caused by the mutation of a prion; and sporadic fatal insomnia, caused by a random mutation of the same prion that causes fatal familial insomnia.

Classic CJD, as researchers now call the original form of Creutzfeldt-Jakob disease, is not the same as vCJD; it is a different form of the disease. Classic CJD has been known to health experts for several decades and appears to occur randomly but rarely (at a rate of about one case per million people each year) in countries throughout the world. Like other TSEs, CJD gradually and progressively destroys brain tissue. There doesn't seem to be a pattern to CJD cases, which occur mainly in older (and even elderly) people. There is some speculation that CJD tends to run in families; research continues to explore this theory. Scientists identified a new form of CJD, which they named variant CJD, in Britain in 1994, and determined it is the disease that infects humans who have consumed BSE-contaminated beef products.

Classic CJD, and variant CJD differ in several key ways (see the table).

DIFFERENCES BETWEEN CLASSIC CJD AND VARIANT CJD

Characteristic	Classic CJD	Variant CJD
Average age of onset	63 years and older	26–28 years
Early symptoms	Uncoordinated and jerky movements (ataxia), weakness impaired speech and swallowing	Sudden and serious psychiatric problems or problems with the senses
Length of illness after onset of symptoms	6 months	13 months
Electroencephalogram activity	Pattern unique to CJD	Pattern different from CJD
Brain findings at autopsy	Spongelike degeneration of brain tissue	Clusters of prion deposits surrounded by spongelike holes
Cause	Random occurrence (most cases) or exposure to materials or substances containing tissues from a person who has the disease, such as through certain transplants and other biomedical treatments	Consumption of BSE-contaminated beef products

BSE and its resulting risk of vCJD has been a wake-up call for health-care professionals and the food industry worldwide, providing frightening evidence of the potentially devastating consequences of a global marketplace. Between 1986 and 2001, about 200,000 cases of BSE had been diagnosed in cows in the United Kingdom (95 percent of all cases), Belgium, Denmark, France, Germany, Ireland, Italy, Luxembourg, Liechtenstein, The Netherlands, Northern Ireland, Portugal, Spain, and Switzerland. Between 1994 and 2001, doctors had diagnosed about 100 cases of vCJD directly related to BSE (all in Europe, except for one case in Hong Kong, in which the woman diagnosed with vCJD had lived in Britain and traveled there several times).

Despite the frightening scenario of vCJD, it's important to remember that the disease (like all TSEs) is extremely rare. Those more than 100 diagnosed cases come from a population of well over 60 million people. Through a focused effort to identify and euthanize animals infected with or exposed to BSE, the UK and other European nations believe they have effectively curtailed the risk of contracting vCJD through beef and beef products (and from other meats and meat products). Though scientists believe the risk of BSE exposure is slim, health experts offer these recommendations to keep it at a minimum:

- Do not buy or eat beef or beef products (or other meats) from other countries unless they have been approved for import into the United States. The USDA bans the import from countries where BSE is known to exist.
- Do not eat organ meats, especially brain, or products manufactured from them. Most such meats, known collectively as offal, are now banned in the United States.
- Follow the CDC guidelines for European travelers, which include foregoing beef altogether, or if you choose to eat beef, buying or eating only muscle meats certified as BSE-free and avoiding ground beef and beef sausage or other sausage products that contain beef or beef by-products.

Most scientists believe the European beef supply now is free from BSE contamination, though the United States continues to ban cattle, cows, beef, and beef products from Europe. Countries in the European Union have implemented strong measures to safeguard their beef supply from BSE. Meat that complies with these measures receives an official stamp of approval. Still, many people who travel in Europe and other parts of the world where BSE is known or suspected to exist choose to avoid beef products as a precaution.

Consumer groups have raised some concern about BSE contamination in beef-based products that use animal-derived substances such as amino acids, glycerol, gelatin, enzymes, and blood. Health officials believe the risk is nominal if not nonexistent, because these products are so highly processed; but they cannot unequivocally rule it out. Scientists do know that different tissues in infected cows harbor different levels of BSE. Brain and spinal cord tissues, for example, have very high concentrations, whereas muscle and connective tissue have so far not recorded any. Though the United States has banned products using beef by-products from Europe, it's virtually impossible to enforce the restriction because many products, such as nutritional supplements, are not subject to inspection. Scientists and health officials became alarmed about the possibility of products slipping through the ban in 2001, when a physician discovered herbal supplements in which the list of ingredients included animal brains, testicles, and other organs banned from import into the United States. It's important to read labels carefully, even on products you might not suspect contain beef by-products. If you're not sure, don't buy.

FOOT AND MOUTH DISEASE

Foot and mouth disease (FMD)—sometimes incorrectly called hoof and mouth disease—is a devastating infection for livestock. To date, only one case of FMD in a person has been documented, in Britain in 1967; a handful of suspected cases in 2001 turned out to be negative. (The common and mild childhood infection known as hand, foot, and mouth disease produces similar but much milder symptoms, goes away in a few days, and is caused by a related, but not the same, virus.) So why all the fuss? Because animals that contract it seldom recover to a point of productivity, and the airborne virus moves so rapidly that it can spread to thousands of animals literally on the next breeze—as well as on the shoes and clothing of people who are in contact with infected animals.

FMD, which is actually a family of seven viruses, is highly contagious and infects ruminants (animals that have multiple stomachs and chew cuds) with cloven (split) hooves: cattle, sheep, goats, pigs, and even deer. It causes oozing sores, which are most prominent around the mouth, and the tissues near the hooves, hence, the name foot and mouth disease. Infected animals stop eating, go lame, and lose muscle tissue and body mass. Milk-producing animals stop giving milk and often develop udder sores that would make it impossible to use any milk they did produce.

There is no treatment for FMD, though it is what medical experts call "self-limiting"—it goes away on its own after running its course. While infected animals can recover (usually in several weeks), they seldom return to a level of health at which they can be considered productive. Recovered animals often suffer from recurring infections such as mastitis (infection of the udder) as well as chronic lameness caused by damage to the tissues around the hooves during the active infection stage of the disease. Animals being raised for meat often fail to regain lost weight and muscle mass, making them considerably smaller than their healthy counterparts and thus less efficient for slaughter. To control the spread of the disease, public health officials typically euthanize animals that contract FMD along with animals that have been exposed to the virus.

Though scientists have not ruled out the potential for a human being to contract FMD, if such an infection were to occur it would not come by consuming contaminated meat products but instead through significant direct contact with infected animals. The few suspected cases that public health officials have investigated involved farmers or slaughterhouse workers who had been in close and extended contact with diseased animals.

The economic loss from an FMD epidemic can be catastrophic, however, not only for farmers and producers but also for entire countries. Widespread euthanasia to control FMD's spread means ranchers must start over with new livestock. Entire breeding and production programs come to a screeching halt. Because FMD spreads so quickly and easily, even animals with no signs of the disease that are within geographic proximity to confirmed cases are put to death as a preventive measure. FMD has a nearly 100 percent infection rate, which means that virtually every animal exposed to the disease will become ill. The virus can survive for weeks; one infected animal sent to a new location for breeding or by sale can infect hundreds or even thousands of other animals before anyone knows it is sick. In one outbreak, infected sheep imported into France from Britain passed FMD on to a herd of dairy cattle, which then exposed other livestock.

The last case of FMD in the United States was in 1929, at which time farmers and USDA officials moved swiftly to curtail its spread by immediately euthanizing the infected animals and implementing stringent quarantines. A 2001 outbreak of FMD in the United Kingdom had more far-reaching consequences, essentially shutting down the beef and dairy industry not only in Britain but also throughout Europe. In the United Kingdom alone, agricultural agents destroyed more than 3 million animals during the outbreak, during which time veterinarians confirmed nearly 1,600 infections. Losses extended well into the millions of dollars. The effects of an FMD outbreak extend for years; there is a six-month disinfecting period following the last confirmed case during which ranchers cannot replace lost livestock. It then takes another one to three years to reach a level of productivity.

The most significant effect FMD has for people—you, the consumer—hits the checkbook, not health. The United States imports more than $2 billion in beef and veal from other countries, and in 1989 banned imports of cattle and beef products from Britain as a safeguard against BSE. Bans on those imports, such as the ones imposed during the 2001 European FMD outbreak, can reduce the availability of beef products in grocery stores and restaurants. Such bans also affect live animals, preventing ranchers from importing cattle and other livestock (including sheep, goats, and pigs) for their breeding programs. The consequences of beef bans vary, though generally produce a net result of somewhat higher prices but not a noticeable shortage.

How Safe Is Your Kitchen?

The good news about food-borne illness is that proper handling, preparation, and cooking can eliminate most risks of infection from eating beef. The primary exceptions are BSE, for which there appears to be no means to destroy the illness-causing agent, and certain carcino-gens. So how safe is your kitchen? A 2000 study revealed that three in four American households fail to follow basic food safety practices. Here's what health experts recommend to help prevent beef-borne ill-nesses from infecting you and your family:

- Keep uncooked beef cold (refrigerated at a temperature below 40°F) or frozen until you're ready to cook it. Buy meat last when shopping and put it in the refrigerator or freezer immediately when you get home.

- Don't season and otherwise prepare beef and then leave it sit-ting on the counter or near the grill. If you are marinating beef, keep it in the refrigerator until you're ready to cook it.

- Follow the safe handling guidelines printed on food packages. Do not purchase beef that is older than the sell-by date and do not cook or eat beef that is older than the use-by date.

- Wash your hands with soap and warm water before and after handling beef and other foods, as well as after touching pets and going to the bathroom.

- Always use separate utensils and preparation surfaces for uncooked and cooked beef and other meats. Keep raw or uncooked beef separate from other foods you are preparing as well from cooked foods. Do *not* use the same knife to cut raw beef and then vegetables or other foods.

- Cook beef thoroughly, to an internal temperature of at least 145°F for steaks and roasts and 160°F for ground beef (ham-burger). Use a meat thermometer; the color of the meat doesn't tell you how hot it is (although pink meat is not hot enough).

- Wash cutting boards first in soapy water and then in a mild bleach solution after use, and rinse with hot water. Thoroughly wash all preparation areas and surfaces with soap and water (or a mild bleach solution) after preparing beef products, including hamburger.

- Cook sausages and hot dogs until they are steaming hot. Thoroughly reheat leftovers, including sausages and hot dogs, until steaming.

■ Don't let cooked meat sit at room temperature for too long. If you are not going to eat cooked meat items right away, be sure they are held at a temperature of at least 140°F until consumption.

Beef and Your Life

The risk of becoming ill with a food-borne infection is higher than most people recognize. The CDC reports that one in four Americans will get a food-borne illness this year. While *you* can reduce your risk by properly handling and preparing beef (as well as other raw meats), you don't have very much control over beef that *others* handle and prepare. When you go out to eat at a restaurant or to a barbecue party, how do you know whether the beef you're eating is safe and pathogen free? You don't. For your health and safety, you must take charge of your choices. While beef isn't inherently bad, there are plenty of reasons to reduce its presence in your diet. Read on for more reasons . . . and for ways to transition to a low- or no-beef way of life.

3

Digestion
and Metabolism

So just what is it about beef that gets people all hyped up about health benefits and risks? How is beef different from any other meat or food that you eat? While you might look at food, including beef, in terms of taste and satisfaction, health experts look at it in terms of nutritional content. During Memorial Day weekend, America's traditional first summer celebration, barbecues all across the country grill more than 60 million pounds of beef. The typical 3.5-ounce, cooked, regular (not lean) ground beef patty—generally served as the infamous sandwich—delivers 287 calories, giving your body 23 grams of protein; 21 grams of fat; and various levels of nutrients such as iron, zinc, vitamin B_6, and vitamin B_{12}.

The truth is, beef is nothing special and is not a benefit to your health if it accounts for too much of your diet. Eating beef can certainly provide your body with valuable nutrients. But it can also give you a fair amount of dietary fat, much of which is saturated, the "bad" fat implicated in many health problems from heart disease to cancer. There are many other foods that are equally, if not more, nutritious than beef. Poultry, fish, whole grains, legumes, nuts, seeds, fruits, and vegetables are rich in the nutrients essential for strong, healthy bodies. They are also lower in saturated fat (the exceptions being coconut or palm oils, which are high in saturated fat), if not all together fat-free. (See Chapter 6 for more on fats.)

Eating beef is really more of a social habit than a dietary necessity, and there are no nutrients in beef that you can't get from other foods. So let's take a look at how your body (not your taste buds!) views beef.

Anatomy Basics: Your Digestive System

Beyond satisfying your taste buds and appetite, the process of eating is the first stage of a complex sequence of events designed to provide your body with the nutrients that serve as its fuel. We call this digestion, from the Latin word *digestus*, meaning to break down" or "decompose." Digestion transforms the food you eat into the nutrients your body needs. To understand what happens after you eat that burger or steak, you need to understand your body's digestive system and how it functions.

Digestion is a mostly mechanical process. The ancient Greek physician Galen (130–200 C.E.) believed that digestion directly produced the body's blood. Although through the centuries other physicians and scientists demonstrated that the connection isn't quite that simple, Galen was on the right track. Digestion is the essence of your body's sustenance; it breaks foods down, reducing them to the elemental substances that your body uses to make, maintain, and repair cells.

OPEN WIDE: THE MOUTH

Open your mouth, and you've opened the entrance to your body's digestive system. Soft, moist tissue lines this cavity, which houses the most powerful muscle in the human body—the tongue—and two rows of harder-than-bone structures, the teeth. Shiny hard enamel coats your teeth, making them stronger than bone and resistant (though not immune) to damage and decay.

Other key structures of your mouth include the lips, palate, cheeks, salivary glands, and pharynx (throat). As you chew (a process known technically as mastication), all of these structures come into play. Carbohydrate digestion begins in the mouth. Protein and fat digestion primarily begins in the stomach. Swallowing pushes the bolus (chewed food) down a muscular tube—your esophagus—to your stomach.

DIGESTIVE POWERHOUSE: THE STOMACH

When food reaches your stomach, the muscles of the stomach churn it every which way to prepare it for its journey through the rest of your digestive system. The stomach resides under the lower left portion of your ribs in the front of your body. It looks like a deeply wrinkled sac when empty and can expand to hold up to 2 quarts (just over 2 liters) after a meal, such as Thanksgiving dinner or an all-you-can-eat prime rib buffet. Your stomach works more efficiently when not stretched to its limit; if you eat just until you feel full instead of until you can't take another bite, your stomach is more likely to contain one-half to two-thirds of its maximum capacity.

Hydrochloric acid mixes with digestive enzymes (such as pepsin and lipase) in the stomach to create a solution that further breaks the food down and turns it into a thick liquid. Under normal circumstances, your stomach begins to produce and release these digestive substances when you first smell or taste food, which trigger sensors in the brain that signal the stomach that food is on the way. The soupy solution that results after this churning and mixing is called chyme. When it reaches the proper consistency, a valve opens at the base of the stomach to let the chyme pour into the small intestine.

THE REAL WORK OF DIGESTION: THE SMALL INTESTINE

Most of the work of digestion takes place in the small intestine, which if stretched out from its coiled and looped posture would measure more than 20 feet in length. Here, enzymes from the pancreas and small intestine, bile from the liver (via the gallbladder), and hormones join the mix to finish breaking down food into its basic components. The small intestine completes the digestion of carbohydrates (converting them to glucose molecules), proteins (converting them to amino acids), and fats or lipids (converting them to fatty acids and glycerol—an extensive process!). When reduced to their most basic structures, these nutrients are then absorbed into the bloodstream through the walls of the small intestine and carried to the parts of the body that need them. Rhythmic, wavelike contractions of the small intestine's muscular wall, called peristalsis, move the chyme along at a steady pace. The food from a typical meal can take 8 to 12 hours to complete its journey through the small intestine.

The more fat the food contains, the harder your body works to digest it. A high-fat meal such as prime rib or a burger stays in your small intestine much longer than a low-fat meal will. Because fat is not water soluble on its own (more on this later), it needs to be put into a state that will enable your enzymes to break it down into molecules that can move through your body. Released in the small intestine, bile acts like a detergent, surrounding the fat molecules, making them soluble. Bile is produced by your liver and then concentrated and stored in your gallbladder. A meal high in fat can pose a challenge to your digestive system if the effort to digest it exceeds the amount of bile your body has stored. If this is the case, some of the fat you eat travels down your intestines incompletely digested. This can be rather uncomfortable, as you can imagine, and is one reason you might experience bloating, gas, and abdominal discomfort after indulging in the bet-you-can't-eat-the-whole-thing 32-ounce super steak at your favorite restaurant. These signs represent a clear message from your digestive system that it is not happy with your food choices.

END OF THE LINE: THE LARGE INTESTINE

From the small intestine, the now mostly digested meal passes into the large intestine (part of which is the colon). The large intestine is much shorter and thicker than the small intestine, about 4 to 5 feet long in an adult and 2 to 3 inches in diameter. The large intestine absorbs some vitamins as well as water. It is also within the large intestine that your body manufactures important nutrients, such as vitamin K. The material that remains consists of substances your body could not digest (including insoluble fiber, undigested food particles, and wastes or by-products of digestion). The large intestine consolidates the waste material as feces (stool), which passes into the rectum for storage until you eliminate it via a bowel movement.

Food Chemistry Basics: Metabolism

From your body's perspective, eating is all about providing the basic metabolic units your body needs to go about its daily activities—the activities that keep you alive not to mention healthy and well. This is, according to your body, the only reason to eat (it's your mind that has other ideas!). Once your digestive system reduces the food you eat to its most basic elements, the chemical processes of metabolism engage. Metabolism exists in two forms, catabolic and anabolic. *Catabolism* is the process of breaking complex compounds into simple substances, and *anabolism* is the process of building simple substances into complex compounds. Most of the chemical activity that takes place during digestion is catabolic.

Your basal metabolic rate (BMR) is the rate at which your body uses energy to fuel all of your body's basic activities needed to keep you alive, such as pumping your heart and inflating (and deflating) your lungs. The amount of energy, or calories, you use in a day is primarily determined by your BMR—roughly 60 percent of your caloric expenditure is from your BMR. Another 10 percent of your caloric expenditure is used to digest the food you eat. How many more calories you expend in a day is determined by your physical activity. Walking a few yards, say, to your car parked in front of your house will increase your caloric expenditure some, but walking a mile around a park will increase your caloric expenditure further. And how many calories you expend in a day determines the amount of calories you can eat to maintain, gain, or lose weight. In general, calories consumed must equal calories expended or you will gain or lose weight accordingly.

Of course, there are many things that come into play with body weight maintenance, such as the amount of body fat or muscle you have. (See Chapter 8 for more on calories and weight management.) When your activity level is low (as when you sit behind a desk all day) your body burns fewer calories, making excess calories available for storage as fat. When your activity level is higher (as you take a brisk 30-minute walk, for example), your body's metabolism revs up and its calorie needs increase.

CARBOHYDRATES: POWER SURGE!

Carbohydrates are your body's (as well as your brain's, but for simplicity we'll consider the mind and body as one here) preferred energy, or calorie, source. We were built primarily to burn carbohydrates as our fuel for life. We need energy not only to accomplish our daily activities but for living itself. All of our bodily systems—from our heart and lungs to our digestive tracts—are like machines that need an energy source to keep them and, therefore, us going. The carbohydrate fuel we use is in the form of glucose. Almost all of the carbohydrates we eat eventually become glucose, which is used to power our bodies.

If you don't have enough glucose in your system, your body compensates. It dips into your carbohydrate reserves, called glycogen (found in the liver and muscle tissue), to make glucose—a simple process. Athletes who carbohydrate load are "stocking the stores" of glycogen in their muscles, so their bodies can draw from them during long competitive events (such as marathons), when food is unavailable.

If your glycogen reserves are empty (as in the case of fasting or when you go longer than a day with too little or no food), your body might be forced to turn to lean tissue—that is, your skeletal muscles and your organs, such as the heart, liver, and lungs—to get protein that will be broken down into amino acids. The amino acids are then used to make glucose. As you can imagine, it isn't a good idea to let your body strip your lean tissues of protein just to make energy. Your body also can break down fat for energy. (See Chapter 8 for more information.)

The carbohydrates we eat come in two forms: simple and complex. Simple carbohydrates, more commonly referred to as simple sugars, are further classified into monosaccharides and disaccharides. The most common monosaccharides are glucose and fructose (the sugar found in fruit). Sucrose, or table sugar, is a disaccharide. Maltose (did some-body say *beer*?) and lactose (the sugar found largely in milk) are also disaccharides.

Complex carbohydrates have longer, more complex chemical struc-tures than simple sugars. Starch, found in plant foods such as whole grains and legumes, is a good example. Your body can easily digest starch. The other important complex carbohydrate is fiber. Fiber, also known as roughage, helps you clean out your system, so to speak, and helps eliminate waste from your body. Fiber has been justly promoted as a health-enhancing food substance. Not only does it clear out waste material but as research indicates, it also helps stave off many chronic diseases such as heart disease and certain cancers. Fiber is found only in plant foods, such as whole grains, legumes, vegetables, fruits, nuts, and seeds.

Beef does not contain any carbohydrates. Therefore, it doesn't pro-vide you with your body's preferred energy source or with disease-fighting fiber. A diet that is largely dominated by beef (as well as other animal meats) usually provides limited complex carbohydrates. As a result, the fiber and important nutrients these foods give us usually fall below recommended guidelines for optimal health. Cutting back or eliminating beef from your diet and incorporating more plant foods will help make your diet more balanced and health promoting.

PROTEIN: BULKING UP

Protein is the primary nutritional reason people eat beef. Beef is considered a high-quality protein because it is a "complete" protein. That is, beef contains the essential amino acids that your body needs to do its work. Essential amino acids are the ones your body cannot man-ufacture; therefore, they are "essential" to have in the diet. But, these amino acids are no more "superior" than the ones the body does make. All animal meats (beef, pork, poultry, and fish, as well as eggs) are con-sidered complete, high-quality protein, so there's nothing magical or special about beef.

An "incomplete" protein doesn't supply all of the essential amino acids that the body needs. This type of protein is found in plant foods, such as legumes (with the exception of the soybean) and whole grains. However, it is easy to make your daily protein, or amino acid, intake complete by eating a wide variety of foods *throughout the day.* Contrary to popular belief, foods in one particular meal do not have to "complement" each other from an amino acid perspective. The key is to eat a wide variety of plant foods throughout the day to provide your body with all of the building blocks it needs to make body protein. If you are planning to follow or are already following a vegetarian diet, consultation with your primary care physician and a registered dietitian helps ensure that your protein (and therefore, amino acid) intake is sufficient for your individual needs.

Protein has many functions within your body. Most important are cell growth and maintenance. Protein can also be used as an energy source. Dietary protein gives your body the material it needs to grow, as well as to make enzymes, hormones, and antibodies (to fight infection). It also helps maintain your body's fluid balance.

Some people eat beef believing that this will give them buff muscles. Wrong! Although your muscles and beef (a cow's muscles) are both made up of protein, the only way to gain muscle mass is to move your muscles or lift heavy objects. And carbohydrates, not proteins, fuel your muscles to do such strength-training activities. So contrary to popular belief, beef is not a magic bullet for gaining muscle mass.

The Recommended Dietary Allowance (RDA) for a typical healthy adult man is about 60 grams of protein; the typical healthy adult woman needs about 50 grams. (Pregnant and lactating women need an additional 10 to 15 grams of protein daily.) Most people can easily obtain the protein they need through a balanced diet.

More is not better when it comes to protein. In fact, too much protein in your diet can lead to health problems. Your body does not store extra protein for future use. Instead, your body either uses the protein as energy or stores it as body fat. Because a diet high in protein is likely to include animal-based foods, such as steak, it is also likely to be high in fat. This means extra calories, which can potentially lead to obesity. Furthermore, protein metabolism requires vitamin B_6, so if you eat more than the recommended amount of protein you run the risk of short-changing your body of this vital nutrient.

Many experts believe that protein intake should be limited to no more than twice your RDA, when enough calories are present in the diet, to avoid possible complications. (See Chapter 5 for detailed information about protein.)

FAT: THE GOOD AND THE BAD

Fat . . . eeewww! Who likes fat? Well, truth be told—we all do. Fat adds flavor and texture to many foods from baked goods to spreads, such as mayonnaise. And despite the bad rap fat gets, a certain level of dietary fat is necessary for your body to function properly. Notice we said "certain" level. This is the critical point about fat consumption. The problem is not that we consume fat but that we Americans tend to consume too much fat—and in the heart-unhealthy saturated form.

Fats are composed of fatty acids that affect health. Just as with amino acids, there are essential and nonessential fatty acids. Essential fatty acids are those that your body needs but cannot manufacture. So it must obtain them through the foods you eat. Nonessential fatty acids are those that your body uses and can manufacture from other substances drawn from your diet during digestion and metabolism.

Fats as we consume them exist in the form of triglycerides. Triglycerides are three fatty acids bounded together by glycerol. When we digest dietary fat, the triglyceride structure is broken down and the individual fatty acids are released. Fatty acids contain carbon, hydrogen, and oxygen and there are basically four kinds, which are delineated by their chemical structures.

Saturated fatty acids have been shown to raise blood cholesterol levels. Eating too much saturated fat, which is found primarily in animal-based foods, such as fatty beef and butter, can increase the risk for heart disease. Saturated fats are often referred to as the "bad" fat.

Polyunsaturated fats have been shown to be neutral in regards to the blood cholesterol and heart disease link. They neither raise nor lower blood cholesterol levels. Sources of polyunsaturated fat include corn and safflower oil. One specific type of polyunsaturated fat is known as omega-3 fatty acids, which are found abundantly in fatty fish and flaxseed. Omega-3 fatty acids appear to protect heart health by helping to prevent blood clots from forming, and to keep the heart pumping at a regular beat.

Monounsaturated fats also have been shown to be quite beneficial for heart health. These fats are often dubbed the "good" fats (along with omega-3 fatty acids). They appear to raise high-density lipoproteins (HDL), which has been linked to a decreased risk of heart disease. Foods high in monounsaturated fat include olive oil, canola oil, and many nuts and seeds.

While a few trans fatty acids occur naturally, most of the ones found in the modern diet are unnaturally created in food processing. When hydrogen is artificially added to an otherwise unsaturated oil (such as corn oil or soybean oil), this forms a strange-looking, more solid, "trans" structure. Creation of a "hydrogenated" or "partially hydrogenated" oil (words you will see listed in the ingredients of many processed foods), extends the shelf life of the food products that contain them. Researchers believe that trans fatty acids can be as bad for your heart as saturated fat.

A little bit of fat in the diet is good—your body clearly needs fat to carry out some of its most important functions. And yes, beef is a source of fat, but the fat in beef is primarily saturated, which is not so good for heart health. (See Chapters 4 and 6 for more on fat and heart disease.) Ideally, we want to eat foods that are limited in saturated fatty acids and instead feature the good fats—monounsaturated (for example, olive oil) and omega-3 fatty acids (in fatty fish). However, even the good fats should be used in moderation to avoid obesity.

VITAMINS AND MINERALS

Vitamins and minerals play vital roles in all of the processes that take place in your body. Many vitamins and minerals help the body's enzymatic processes run smoothly, thereby keeping us healthy and alive. Vitamins and minerals also play a role in:

■ Keeping bones strong (calcium, magnesium, vitamin D)
■ Keeping red blood cells intact (folate, vitamin B_{12})
■ Keeping immune function strong (vitamin C)
■ Maintaining optimal vision (vitamin A)
■ Fighting dangerous free radicals (vitamin E)
■ Synthesizing blood-clotting proteins (vitamin K)
■ Maintaining proper fluid balance within the body (sodium, potassium)

Indeed, vitamins and minerals are essential for health and life. Except for vitamin D, which your body can manufacture when exposed to sunlight, the vitamins and minerals your body needs are all essential—your body must get them through the foods you eat.

There are two categories of vitamins: water soluble and fat soluble. The water-soluble vitamins are vitamin C and the B vitamins—thiamine (B_1), riboflavin (B_2), niacin, pantothenic acid, pyridoxine (B_6), biotin, folic acid, and cyanocobalamin (B_{12}). The fat-soluble vitamins are vitamins A, D, E, and K.

Water-Soluble Vitamins

The water-soluble vitamins dissolve in water-based fluids. They are transported easily in your bloodstream to where they are needed in your body. Once your body has enough of these vitamins, any extra quantities are excreted. Your body cannot store excess water-soluble vitamins for future use but must instead replenish its supply in accordance with its needs.

Those who want to reduce or eliminate beef from their diets might be concerned about getting enough of water-soluble vitamin B_{12}. Yes, beef is a good source of vitamin B_{12}, but it is not the only source, nor is it particularly the *best* source. Sardines and tuna contain more vitamin B_{12} than, say, ground beef. Other foods, such as cottage cheese, yogurt, shrimp, haddock, and eggs also contain ample amounts of the vitamin. Even those who decide to consume a diet that is without any animal meats, eggs, or dairy products can get enough vitamin B_{12} through fortified soy beverages and/or supplements.

Fat-Soluble Vitamins

Fat-soluble vitamins can dissolve only in lipids (fats). Therefore, they must be attached to fat-containing substances in your body to be transported to the tissues that need them. This is one of the reasons why you need *some* fat in your diet—to make the fat-soluble vitamins available to your body. Your body stores excess quantities of fat-soluble vitamins in your fat tissues. Because of this, fat-soluble vitamins can accumulate to levels that become toxic. It's especially important not to exceed the daily recommended amounts unless your doctor instructs you otherwise.

Minerals

Minerals are other chemicals your body needs for health. The major minerals—those needed in quantities of about 1 gram or so per day in the diet (unless otherwise prescribed by your doctor)—include calcium, magnesium, potassium, sodium, phosphorus, chloride, and sulfur. The trace minerals are generally needed in smaller amounts and include iron, zinc, iodine, copper, fluoride, selenium, chromium, molybdenum, manganese, and cobalt.

Most people can obtain the minerals and vitamins they need through the foods they eat; supplements are not necessary for healthy adults who eat balanced diets. Beef is a relatively good source of vitamins—such as vitamin B_6, and vitamin B_{12}—and minerals—such as iron and zinc—that your body needs to stay healthy. These vital nutrients are abundant in other foods, however, so beef is not the *only* source for them.

4

High Beef Consumption and Your Health

There is considerable debate about the relationship between beef and health. While some correlations are clear, such as that between saturated fat and heart disease, others are ambiguous. One challenge is trying to sort out the roles of the many variables. Is it the beef or is it the couch-potato lifestyle? Scientists have identified daily exercise as having an important influence on many health conditions. And because beef is generally high in calories from fat, people whose diets include hefty portions of beef often are overweight or obese. Is it the beef or is it the body fat? Obesity itself has an effect on many health conditions. (See Chapter 8 for more on body weight.) While there remains much for scientists to learn about the role nutrition plays in health and in disease, research over the past few decades has provided a great many insights that you can use to safeguard and improve your health.

Beef and Heart Disease

Heart disease is the leading cause of death among Americans over age 30, claiming more than 900,000 lives each year—nearly 2 Americans die every minute from heart disease. And more than 60 million Americans live with some form of heart disease—that's 1 in 5 people. Researchers at the Centers for Disease Control and Prevention (CDC) project that by eliminating the major forms of heart disease, we could extend the life expectancy of the average American by seven years!

There are many forms of heart disease. Some arise from specific physical conditions such as rheumatic fever. Lifestyle matters such as diet and exercise do not influence these types. Most forms of heart disease, however, *are* linked to lifestyle. And the connection is strong for coronary heart disease (CHD), cardiovascular disease (CVD), hypertension (high blood pressure), and stroke (cerebrovascular disease). Eating a diet heavy in beef may contribute to a variety of lifestyle characteristics that play a role in heart disease.

Many factors determine whether and how heart disease develops. Some of these are absolute or fixed risks—circumstances that are beyond your ability (or your doctor's) to change. Other risks are relative or mutable—circumstances that are within your ability to change.

Researchers have identified three major fixed risks for heart disease:

- **Age.** Everyone's risk of heart disease increases with age, regardless of other risk factors.
- **Gender.** Men have a higher risk of developing heart disease, especially at earlier ages, than women.
- **Heredity (genetic predisposition).** Your odds of developing heart disease increase several-fold if other members of your family (particularly your parents or siblings) have or had heart disease. Many researchers consider family history to be the most significant risk factor for heart disease. Furthermore, the American Heart Association (AHA) and many other researchers include race in this risk factor; African Americans and Hispanics, for example, have a significantly higher rate of heart disease than white Americans.

Having one or more fixed risk (and we all have at least one—the age factor) makes it even more important for you to do what you can to control your mutable risk factors. Mutable risk factors for heart disease, factors you can influence positively by changing your behavior, include the following:

■ **Tobacco use.** The leading disease risk of cigarette smoking is not cancer but heart disease. Smoking damages the arteries, causing them to stiffen and become less flexible; it accounts for one in five deaths from CVD.

■ **Sedentary lifestyle.** A sedentary lifestyle encourages too much sitting. Not getting enough physical activity contributes to high blood lipid levels (cholesterol and triglycerides), high blood pressure, and excess body weight.

■ **High blood lipid levels.** Fatty deposits can line your blood vessels, causing them to become narrow and stiff. (See Chapter 6 for more information about dietary and blood lipids.)

■ **Excess body weight and obesity.** Extra body fat contributes to a wide range of health conditions and often coexists with problems such as high blood lipid levels.

A risk that straddles the line between absolute and relative risk is diabetes mellitus. Diabetes is a disease in which insulin does not fully transport glucose from the bloodstream, leading to dangerously high levels of blood sugar. Having diabetes increases your risk for heart disease. Lifestyle is not a contributing factor for developing type 1 diabetes (sometimes called juvenile onset), which develops when the pancreas stops producing insulin. Health experts do consider lifestyle to be a factor for type 2 diabetes (sometimes called adult onset), however. Type 2 diabetes is usually a disease of insulin resistance rather than an inability to produce insulin (your pancreas produces insulin, but your cells can't use it properly and consequently can't use glucose properly either). About 90 percent of the 16 million Americans (and 135 million people worldwide) who have type 2 diabetes are overweight or obese. Lifestyle changes—such as improving the diet; starting an exercise program; and achieving healthy, sustained weight loss—are often successful in controlling type 2 diabetes and so reduce the overall heart disease risk.

A diet high in beef contributes to or exacerbates all of the mutable risks, except tobacco use, for heart disease. This means you can lower several risks for heart disease at the same time just by reducing or eliminating the beef you eat. Although it's not within the scope of this book to discuss tobacco use or exercise, we urge you to address these factors in your life if they are relevant. If you smoke or otherwise use tobacco, stop—there are no known health benefits that result from tobacco use . but there is an abundance of potential health problems.

And, as the AHA emphasizes: Get moving! Adults need a minimum of 30 to 40 minutes of physical activity at least three to four days a week—and this doesn't include shuffling around the living room looking for the remote control—for overall health and well-being. You can take your exercise all at once or in short segments throughout the day, as long as it adds up. And now, back to beef.

BEEF, HOMOCYSTEINE, AND YOUR HEART

Homocysteine is a natural amino acid waste product that your body makes when metabolizing the essential fatty acid methionine. Methionine is found in red meat, such as beef. Homocysteine is used in your body to help maintain and grow tissue. If more homocysteine is in your system than your body needs, your body converts homocysteine back into methionine or other amino acids that will be eliminated in the urine. To drive this conversion, your body needs folate (found in legumes, oranges, and leafy dark greens), vitamin B_{12} (found in tuna, cottage cheese, and fortified whole grains), and vitamin B_6 (found in potatoes, watermelon, and bananas) to be present.

If an excessive amount of homocysteine is circulating in the blood—which potentially can occur from a diet that is high in beef and low in folate, the body's normal mechanisms of eliminating homocysteine are overwhelmed. Although beef is a good source of vitamin B_{12} and vitamin B_6, it is not a rich source of folate. All of these B vitamins need to be present to eliminate homocysteine from the body. Researchers have found that people with high levels of homocysteine in their blood have an increased risk of atherosclerosis, or hardening of the arteries, which can lead to a heart attack or stroke.

Many experts hope that homocysteine will be checked in people as often as blood cholesterol is checked, as a means of monitoring the risk of heart disease. For now, the AHA recommends that people who have risk factors for heart disease have their homocysteine levels monitored. Eating a diet that will provide ample amounts of folate, vitamin B6, and vitamin B12 (preferably through plant foods and fish), and that is low in red meat comsumption, can help prevent an elevated homocysteine level.

THE SATURATED FAT CONNECTION

More than 40 million Americans have blood cholesterol levels that exceed the levels researchers believe to be healthy. People with high cholesterol have twice the risk for heart attack than people have healthy levels. The most significant dietary source of lipids in terms of blood cholesterol levels is saturated fat. And much of the saturated fat in the typical American diet comes from—you guessed it—beef (although all animal-based foods contain some amount of saturated fat).

The AHA recommends that no more than 7 to 10 percent of your diet come from saturated fat. For a daily diet that contains 2,000 calories, this is equal to 15 (7 percent) to 20 (10 percent) grams of saturated fat (1 gram of fat has 9 calories). But the typical American diet gets 20 to 30 percent of its daily calories from fat. When you look at what happens when beef is the centerpiece of a meal, it's easy to see why this is the case. A 3-ounce (cooked) lean hamburger patty has 6 grams of saturated fat. Add a 1-ounce slice of cheese (Cheddar or American, 6 grams saturated fat), 1 tablespoon of mayonnaise (2 grams saturated fat), and a bun (1 gram saturated fat), and you're already at 15 grams of saturated fat—7 percent.

So do you have to give up beef entirely to lower the amount of saturated fat you consume? No (although the delicious recipes given later in the book will entice you to do just that if you haven't already made the decision). But you do need to recognize how significant the saturated fat content is in the beef you choose to eat. It's also important to increase the amounts of other foods that you eat, especially those that add fiber such as vegetables, legumes, fruits, and whole grains. It is believed that fiber absorbs a certain amount of dietary fat, keeping your body from digesting it. Foods that are high in fiber can also help you to feel full, reducing your urge to snack or fill up on high-fat alternatives like a second burger. The AHA recommends that people get 25 to 30 grams of fiber a day.

THE FATTY FACTS OF HEART DISEASE

When you eat foods that are high in saturated fat, such as beef, you run the risk of elevating your total blood cholesterol by raising a particular type of blood cholesterol, known as low-density lipoprotein (LDL). LDL is a "transport" vehicle in the body that carries cholesterol to the cells. Cells use cholesterol for many things. If too much LDL is circulating in your blood, there is an increased risk that some of these vehicles will oxidize along the walls of the arteries that carry blood to your cells. This oxidation reaction damages the walls of the arteries. The damaged area of the artery wall will then no longer be completely smooth, and plaque (or fatty deposits) will begin to accumulate.

Over time, the plaque can build up and clog the arteries, slowing the flow of blood through them. The artery walls may also become stiff (called arteriosclerosis), which prevents the vessels from contracting and relaxing, as they need to do to move your blood through your body. These circumstances increase the strain on your heart, as it tries to pump blood through your narrowed arteries, which also causes your blood pressure to rise.

The higher pressure of the blood flowing through the restricted channels increases the likelihood that a chunk of the gunk clogging your arteries might dislodge (think of partially kinking a hose to increase its spraying pressure). This floating debris becomes an embolus (a thrombus if it's a clot) that could short-circuit your brain (stroke) or cut off blood to your heart (heart attack).

The steak you grilled for dinner last night isn't going to cause a stroke or heart attack tomorrow or even next week. The process of plaque buildup in the arteries takes years if not decades. Some researchers believe it is a process that can start in childhood, which is good reason to establish healthy eating habits in your kids while they are young. (See Chapter 10 for tips.) Fortunately, your efforts to halt and even reverse this process can have a relatively quick effect.

There is much researchers still don't know about the relationship between diet and heart disease, but one thing they know for certain: Diet makes a difference. What you eat might not go straight to your heart, but eventually it affects everything that matters to your heart. Reducing the amount of saturated fat that you eat can lower the levels of low-density lipoproteins (LDLs) in blood. Increasing the amount of plant foods (vegetables, legumes, and fruits) in your diet will provide you with an arsenal of antioxidants that will help prevent LDL from oxidizing. A diet rich in plant-based foods will also provide you with fiber and phytochemicals (more on this later), which have been shown to be protective against heart disease. Focusing on monounsaturated fats (found in olive oil and many nuts and seeds) as your principle source of fat will help to increase your level of high-density lipoproteins (HDLs), the "good" cholesterol. HDL is considered to be "good" because it is involved with eliminating cholesterol from the body. Adding regular physical activity (such as walking 30 minutes a day, four days a week) to the picture further improves your blood cholesterol levels by helping to raise HDL.

Beef and Cancer

Cancer is the second-leading cause of death in the United States, claiming more than 550,000 lives each year—about 1,500 lives lost each day. And each year, more than 1.2 million people will find out that they have cancer—40 percent of whom will not survive five years. Yet many health experts believe that lifestyle changes—such as diet and exercise—could eliminate as many as 70 percent of cancers.

Research shows that populations in which the traditional diet is high in plant foods, such as vegetables and fruits, and low in red meat have a significantly lower rate of certain cancers (especially cancers affecting the digestive system) compared to populations whose diets are the reverse. This has led to speculation that red meat causes cancer. So far, there is no research that supports this assertion. However, there is considerable research that supports an association between cooked meat and carcinogens, establishing a link between beef and cancer.

Carcinogens are chemicals that cause cancer. Researchers have identified a number of carcinogens in beef that is cooked to very well done and especially when it is charred, as often occurs during grilling and frying. The lipids in meat (its fats) oxidize as the meat cooks. The chemical changes that take place during cooking create substances called mutagens (substances that promote mutations). Among the mutagens that form when beef cooks are heterocyclic amines (HCAs). The higher the cooking temperature, the more HCAs that form.

HCAs are known animal carcinogens—that is, researchers know they cause cancer in laboratory animals. What they don't know is exactly what happens to HCAs when they enter the human body or what stimulates their carcinogenic actions. Some researchers believe that HCAs somehow become activated and accumulate in body tissues that are sensitive to them, such as breast tissue. How this might happen remains a mystery. Other scientists believe that because beef stays in your digestive system for a relatively long time, compared to other foods, it results in repeated and prolonged contact with HCAs. This sets up the tissue changes that eventually become cancer.

These findings about HCA raise a dilemma for beef-eaters. On the one hand, health experts recommend cooking beef thoroughly to kill any pathogens that might be present. On the other hand, doing so releases chemicals that are suspected of causing cancer. The best solution is . . . Beef Busters! If beef is not part of your diet, this is not a dilemma for you. (Note: Researchers also have been investigating HCA formation in the charring of other meats, such as pork. Try not to overcook any type of meat to the point of causing a charred appearance.)

SATURATED FAT AND CANCER

Potential carcinogens aren't the only cancer risk of a diet high in red meats. Once again, the hazards of saturated fat return to haunt your health. There is a strong connection between a diet high in fat, especially saturated fat, and some forms of colon cancer, breast cancer, and prostate cancer. Researchers also know that there is a correlation between excess body weight and the risk for these same cancers—and that a high-fat diet is a leading factor in obesity.

As is the case with heart disease, cancer risks are either absolute (fixed) or relative (mutable). Risks vary according to the kind of cancer; but, in general, the fixed risks for cancer include the following:

- **Age.** Your risk of developing cancer increases as you grow older.
- **Heredity (genetic predisposition).** You are more likely to develop certain forms of cancer if other members of your family have (or have had) them.
- **Intestinal polyps or chronic inflammatory bowel disease.** People with these medical conditions are more likely to develop colon cancer.
- **Menopause (women).** Estrogen levels drop off after menopause. A postmenopausal woman's risk for breast cancer and uterine cancer increases.

The risk factors for cancer that you can change, the mutable risks, are similar to those for heart disease:

- **Tobacco use.** Tobacco use, especially cigarette smoking, increases your risk for cancer not only of the lungs, but also of the lips, mouth, throat, stomach, pancreas, colon, and rectum, among others.
- **Sedentary lifestyle.** Regular exercise has the potential to help prevent or even slow cancer.
- **A diet high in animal-based foods.** People whose primary food sources are animal based have a significantly higher risk for

developing colorectal cancer than people who depend on plant-based foods. There is also evidence that a meat-heavy diet increases the risk for breast, prostate, and stomach cancers.

The American Cancer Society (ACS) estimates that one-third of the cancers that result in death each year are directly attributable to diet. Research studies implicate a meat-based diet as a contributing factor in colorectal cancer and prostate cancer and possibly endometrial (uterine) cancer and breast cancer. Much research done on prostate cancer suggests that there is a correlation between saturated fat in the diet and increased testosterone levels in a man's body. Researchers believe this is the result of the fatty acids alpha-linolenic acid and arachidonic acid, which the body produces as it digests meat. These fatty acids increase a man's blood testosterone level, which has the effect of turbo-charging the growth of prostate cancer cells. There is speculation that a similar process occurs with breast cancer and endometrial (uterine) cancer, although the research is not as conclusive.

REDUCE YOUR RISK FOR CANCER: CUT OUT THE BEEF

As with heart disease, we encourage you to stop smoking and start exercising if these risk factors apply to you. And we assume that if you're reading this book, your diet is high in animal-based foods. Cutting back the amount of beef that you eat, of course, is the first and most significant step for you to take to reduce this risk factor for cancer.

The second, and some researchers believe equally important, step toward reducing your risk for cancer is to add an abundance of plant-based foods to your diet. ACS guidelines call for Americans to choose the majority of the foods they eat from plant sources, a recommendation that supports both reducing meat and increasing other foods that appear to have cancer-fighting qualities. When beef fills your plate, there's not much room left for the vegetables, whole grains, legumes (including soy), nuts and seeds, and fruit that health experts recommend that you eat. This may cause a lack of some nutrients, which some researchers believe is the main culprit (not actual fat intake) for setting the stage for health problems such as heart disease and cancer.

"FIVE A DAY" TO KEEP CANCER AWAY

In 1991 the National Cancer Institute launched an aggressive campaign to educate consumers about the role of diet in preventing cancer, encouraging people to eat at least five servings of fruits and vegetables a day. The ACS and the Food and Drug Administration (FDA) concur with this recommendation. And five a day has become an element of the FDA's dietary guidelines for adults. Researchers say that achieving this one goal can reduce your risk for colorectal cancer, the fourth most common form of cancer in the United States, by as much as 60 percent.

Cancer experts warn that while reducing the amount of red meat you eat or switching to a meat-free lifestyle and increasing the amounts of plant foods you eat (such as vegetables, fruits, legumes, and whole grain products) can significantly reduce your risk for cancer, these measures do not guarantee that you will not get colorectal cancer or other cancers that have been linked to dietary fat. It is still important to see your doctor regularly for health checkups and cancer screenings, and seek help if you develop any suspicious symptoms.

Beef and Obesity

Beef, by itself, does not cause obesity. No food does. But eating too much beef, especially the higher fat cuts of beef can potentially cause weight gain. Typically fat accounts for around a third of beef's weight but almost half of its calories (this varies according to the cut of beef). Gram for gram, a serving of beef is higher in calories than is a serving of food from almost any other food category except sugars and sweets. Many people who are overweight or obese eat diets in which beef takes center plate.

Health experts recommend that no more than 20 to 30 percent of your daily calories come from fat, and no more than 7 to 10 percent of your calories come from saturated fat as part of your total fat intake. The typical American diet is 40 percent fat, although this appears to be dropping as we become more aware of the health consequences of high-fat eating habits. It's entirely possible to meet or exceed your Recommended Dietary Allowance (RDA) of fat (especially saturated fat) in a single beef-based meal (remember that cheeseburger described earlier in this chapter?).

A secondary factor in regard to the calorie content of beef is serving size. While nutritionists view a serving size of cooked beef as 3.5 ounces, a lot of people actually eat servings that are considerably larger. In restaurants, for example, it's nearly impossible to order a steak that is smaller than 8 ounces (about 6 or 7 ounces cooked, depending on how lean the cut is) and many are 12 to 16 ounces (10 to 12 ounces cooked, depending on leanness) or larger. This give you not only far more fat (total and saturated) than the recommendation from the ACS but significantly more calories too. And as you know, your body packs those calories away as body fat.

A 2001 study suggests that obesity has surpassed tobacco use in the United States when it comes to lifestyle habits that are linked to health problems. Your risk of many conditions—such as cancer, type 2 diabetes, and heart disease—goes up as your body weight does. While certainly there are many factors involved in weight management, diet and exercise are the two that you can control. (See Chapter 8 for helpful tips.)

Beef and Other Health Concerns

In addition to increasing your risk for heart disease and cancer, eating beef also raises other health concerns. Food-borne illnesses, as discussed in Chapter 2, remain a significant health concern. Fortunately, you can prevent most of these by following safe meat-handling procedures: Wash your hands and all preparation areas with soap and warm water before and after handling meat; use separate utensils and surfaces for preparing raw meat and any other foods, including cooked meat; and always cook meat to the recommended temperature.

There has been some concern about contracting variant Creutzfeldt-Jakob disease (vCJD) from food supplements that use beef by-products from other countries. So far there are no documented cases of this happening, and health officials in the United States feel confident that embargoes on such products will eliminate this risk. However, there have been discoveries of such supplements because the beef by-products were not clearly noted on the labels. It is important to read labels carefully—and if in doubt, don't buy or use any supplement product containing beef by-products, especially those manufactured abroad.

Bust Your Craving for High-Fat Flavor

Yes, fat adds flavor and texture to foods. Most beef lovers prefer cuts of beef that are marbled with fat, because they've learned to think of them as the most flavorful. It takes your taste buds about two weeks to adjust to the new lower-fat taste, so be sure to give yourself at least that before deciding that you just can't live without the old taste. And once you've gone low fat, you will be surprised to discover that if you eat a high-fat food again, it won't taste as good as you remembered. In fact, you may not like it at all!

If you're feeling a bit overwhelmed by the prospect of making such changes in your lifestyle, relax! We're not going to offer suggestions and then leave you on your own to figure out how to change your lifestyle. Chapter 11, for example, takes you through a step-by-step process for reducing and eliminating beef from your diet. Chapter 12 tells you how to plan delicious and nutritious meals—without beef. And the last four chapters of the book feature recipes that are easy to fix and a delight to eat. The recipes in Chapter 13 help you choose the leanest cuts of beef and eat smaller portions of them, and those in Chapter 14 help you select tasty and nutritious substitutes for beef. Chapter 15 shows you how to add a wider variety of foods to your meals so you can further reduce the amount beef that you eat. And Chapter 16 shows you how you can dine without eating beef at all!

5

Protein and Iron

Protein and iron. These are two nutritional reasons why people eat beef. Yes, protein and iron are vital to human health. And yes, beef is a source for these substances. But beef is not the only source, and it should not be your primary source—for either. Many people worry that they won't get enough of vital nutrients such as protein and iron if they cut back on beef or eliminate it from their diets. But remember—as you are reducing beef, you should be adding a variety of other foods to your diet (later chapters provide tasty and nutritious ways for you to do this). A well-balanced diet (even a vegetarian one) will provide your body with enough protein and iron to function at its best.

A concern many people overlook is the risk of getting *too much* of certain nutrients such as protein and iron. This can have some negative health consequences, which we discuss a bit later in this chapter. But first, let's explore how protein and iron contribute to good health.

Protein and Your Body

Protein is one of the most highly respected nutrients in our diet. It comes from the Greek word *proteios*, which means "of prime importance." Every function of your body requires protein in some way, and every cell contains protein. Proteins form the basis of enzymes, hormones, and other important chemicals in your body. Proteins also form the basis of the antibodies that protect you from illness and infection. Protein is used to build and repair cells and body tissues. (This is no small task—each minute of every day a healthy adult body makes 300 million new cells to replace the 300 million cells that die, maintaining a constant number of cells throughout adult life.) The DNA, or genetic code, in each cell provides the instructions for how the cell assembles its amino acid chains into proteins.

Scientists believe it is a mutated prion, a protein-like agent, that causes variant Creutzfeldt-Jakob disease (vCJD)—the human form of mad cow disease. (See Chapter 2 for more on vCJD.) And they suspect that further research is likely to show that mutated proteins contribute to far more diseases than we now know to be the case. If we eat meat contaminated with bovine spongiform encephalopathy (BSE, or mad cow disease), we are also ingesting the mutated prions, which could re-form in our protein structures, mutating them.

THE MANY CONFIGURATIONS OF PROTEIN

Although we talk about protein as though it were a single substance, there are actually thousands of protein structures. Each has a unique chemical configuration and name, and each serves a specific purpose. Protein comes from various food sources, and the protein that you eat doesn't directly or automatically become protein in your body. Digestion breaks down the proteins in foods into their basic components, which your body then rebuilds into the protein structures that it needs. These basic components, often referred to as building blocks, are called amino acids. The process of joining them into proteins is called protein synthesis.

There are 20 amino acids that combine in various ways to make the 10,000 or so proteins that can exist in just a single cell within your body—similar to the way that the 26 letters in our alphabet can combine to form an almost endless set of words. Amino acids form structures called polypeptide chains—just as letters combine to form words. Polypeptide chains then unite in various ways to become proteins—as words combine to form sentences.

There are two kinds of amino acids, essential and nonessential. Essential amino acids are ones we must get through the foods we eat; our bodies cannot manufacture them. The 9 essential amino acids are histidine, isoleucine, leucine, lysine, methionine, phenylalanine, threonine, tryptophan, and valine. Nonessential amino acids are those that your body can build for you, although your diet should also provide them to ensure there are enough amino acids around for your body to do its work. The 11 nonessential amino acids are alanine, arginine, aspartic acid, cysteine, cystine, glutamic acid, glutamine, glycine, proline, tyrosine, and serine. Some of these, such as glutamine, are considered "conditionally essential" because, under some conditions, the body cannot form enough of them and they must be augmented by diet.

Beef, like all meats, contains all the essential amino acids your body needs. This makes it a "complete" protein. This has given beef an undeserved reputation as the ideal source for protein. Other animal-based foods—such as poultry, fish, eggs, milk, cheese—provide all the essential proteins as well. Soybean-based foods are also considered to be sources of complete protein. (See Chapter 9 for more on soy.) Three ounces of cooked chicken or turkey provide the same amount of protein as 3 ounces of cooked lean beef—about 21 grams. And 1 cup of cooked firm tofu delivers about 19 grams of high-quality protein. (The actual amounts depend on preparation.) All are comparable, when considering protein content.

Eating soy has many advantages in addition to providing a source of complete protein. Generally low in calories and high in fiber, soy has been shown to help reduce the risk of heart disease. Soy-based foods are a rich source of isoflavones, phytochemicals scientists believe fight and might even prevent certain forms of cancer. And soy products appear to reduce many of the discomforts of menopause, such as hot flashes and night sweats.

Incomplete does not mean inadequate or substandard when it comes to protein. It simply means that the food source does not contain all nine essential amino acids. It's not necessary for you to get all the essential amino acids your body needs from a single protein source. If you eat a balanced diet, such as the Beef Buster meal plan, you will get all the amino acids you need for good health.

HOW MUCH PROTEIN DO YOU NEED?

How much protein you need depends on your age (infants and children need more protein than adults because they are growing), your health status (people healing from surgery or from burn wounds, for example, need more protein to help their bodies replenish damaged cells), or whether you are pregnant or lactating (protein is needed to support the growing fetus or to produce milk). In general, however, the average healthy adult doesn't need a whole lot of daily protein to meet his or her needs. For a healthy adult man, the Recommended Dietary Allowance (RDA)—the amount health experts have determined is ideal for optimal health—is about 60 grams of protein a day. For an average healthy adult woman, the RDA is about 50 grams.

It really doesn't take much to meet these amounts. Say you start your day with a bowl of wheat bran cereal (about 1½ cups) and low-fat milk (1 cup). This gives you about 14 grams of protein. Slice a banana over your cereal for added flavor, and you've added 0.5 gram of protein. Round out your morning fare with a slice of whole wheat toast with 1 tablespoon of peanut butter (without any added hydrogenated oils or preservatives), and you add about 6.5 grams more, for a breakfast total of 21 grams of protein.

How about lunch? Tuna on rye is a nutritious choice. Put 3 ounces of tuna between two slices of rye bread and you have about 28 grams of protein. Add a side salad that contains about ½ cup of dark green lettuce, a slice of tomato, and 2 tablespoons of green peas, and you'll add another 1 gram of protein. This already puts you at 50 grams of protein for the day—and your day is just half over! For women, you've met your total RDA for protein, and men, you are just about there.

As you can see, a balanced diet—with or without beef—can easily meet your protein needs. In fact, most Americans consume considerably higher amounts of protein (about 90 grams a day). The best way to know your individual protein needs is to consult with a registered dietitian. Here are some common foods and their protein contents:

- Tempeh (½ cup)—16 grams protein
- Tofu, raw, firm (½ cup)—19 grams protein
- Chicken breast (3 ounces cooked)—26 grams protein
- Turkey breast (3 ounces cooked)—25 grams protein
- Salmon (3 ounces cooked)—23 grams protein
- Tuna (3 ounces cooked)—22 grams protein
- Cottage cheese (1 cup)—28 grams protein
- Egg (1 large)—6 grams protein
- Beef, ground, regular (3 ounces cooked)—23 grams protein

THE HAZARDS OF HIGH-PROTEIN DIETS

You've probably been hearing a lot about high-protein diets lately, with all of the purported health benefits of following such a regimen. What's all of the hoopla about? Well, in general, many of these high-protein diets claim that if the majority of your daily caloric intake comes from foods that are high in protein—most notably animal-based foods such as steak and cheese—and you severely limit carbohydrate foods—including whole grains—then an oasis of health benefits is yours. From quickly losing weight to improving your sex drive, you can have it all if you load up on saturated fat and cholesterol-rich foods. Forget what the American Heart Association, the American Cancer Society, the American Dietetic Association, and just about every other credible health organization recommend about getting enough fiber, vitamins, minerals, phytochemicals, and antioxidants (found primarily in carbohydrate-rich plant foods) to fend off chronic disease and maintain an ideal weight.

Many people are, understandably, drawn to the promise of quick weight loss with these high-protein diets. Who likes to "diet"? Well, dieting is exactly what you are doing on these high-protein regimens that require you to cut calories severely and completely eliminate foods that you have probably enjoyed throughout your life. Even otherwise highly regarded nutritious foods are black listed on these high-protein diets—bananas, carrots, whole-grain breads, and potatoes. The lists of "bad" foods for these diets are amazing!

Indeed, by greatly restricting calories, you will lose weight— quickly. This will happen on any low-calorie diet, whether it's high carbohydrate or high protein. But quick weight loss usually means two things: a loss of body fluids, or water, and a loss of precious lean tissue (such as muscle). So, the diminished numbers on your bathroom scale don't necessarily mean you've lost unwanted body fat.

Even though the thought of eating steak and eggs for breakfast (with no hash browns or toast, mind you), then ham and cheese (with no bread) for lunch, and then prime rib (with no accompanying side dish like rice) may sound tempting at first glance, this kind of diet can really be tolerated only for so long. Remember, your body's preferred energy source is carbohydrates. And without many carbohydrates around, your body shifts into "starvation" and ketosis modes. (See Chapter 8 for more on ketosis.) This is not exactly a state you want to be in if you want to lead an energetic life.

Popular high-protein diets are not as glorious as they seem or as healthy as they proclaim. Following such a diet for an extended time can increase your risk for a number of health problems. One big concern is that many of the high-protein diets are lacking in vitamins and minerals (not to mention fiber), mostly because they restrict plant foods, such as whole grains and fruits. Another reason is that they generally are low in calories, so eating enough of the allowed foods may not cover your vitamin and mineral needs. And even if you were able to get enough of say, calcium, the long-term risk of getting osteoporosis would still be there from eating a high-protein diet, particularly one that almost exclusively features animal meats such as beef.

Researchers at the University of California at San Francisco recently conducted a study that showed women over the age of 65 years whose dietary protein came primarily from animal sources had lower bone density than women whose dietary protein came primarily from plant-based foods. (Lower bone density is linked to osteoporosis and bone fractures.) Other experts believe that eating too much animal protein can increase the risk of osteoporosis based on an excess phosphorus intake. Your body needs to maintain a certain ratio of calcium to phosphorus. Meat is naturally high in phosphorus, so if you eat a lot of beef, you get a lot of phosphorus. To counterbalance the excess phosphorus, your body might take calcium from your bones to maintain the proper ratio between these two substances in the rest of your body.

Another concern with long-term high-protein diets is the increased risk of kidney damage. Although there has been some debate over this issue, eating too much protein does increase the workload of the kidneys, which need to filter the by-products produced from protein metabolism. Overtaxing the kidneys over a long period of time can potentially lead to an increased risk of kidney damage.

And there are issues of an increased risk of heart disease. These high-protein diets claim that foods high in saturated fat, such as beef, are "good" foods that can be eaten at will. Unfortunately, such a diet might lead to an increase in blood cholesterol levels. The corresponding lack of plant foods severely limits fiber, antioxidants, and phytochemical intake, all of which have been found to help stave off the threat of (or to help treat already existing) heart disease.

Even infants and children who are growing rapidly and who certainly need ample amounts of protein in their diets to meet their needs don't benefit from having an extreme excess of dietary protein. In fact, research is under way to determine how much protein can be too much in a child or infant's diet. Health experts are concerned that high protein diets can be harmful for infants and children.

PROTEIN AND AMINO ACID SUPPLEMENTS

What about athletes who push their bodies to perform under extreme circumstances? Do they need dietary supplements to build the muscle mass their sports require? While such supplements are readily available, there is no evidence that they do anything a healthy human body couldn't do with an adequate diet. Healthy adults don't need protein or amino acid supplements. You can get as much protein as your body needs by eating a balanced diet.

Iron and Beef: Heme and Nonheme Iron Sources

Iron is an important dietary mineral that is involved in transporting oxygen from your lungs to the tissues of your body. Your body needs iron to manufacture the hemoglobin in red blood cells that carries oxygen throughout your body. Without enough iron in your diet, your body ends up short on red blood cells and hemoglobin—a health condition called iron-deficiency anemia.

As with protein, beef has been associated as being a superior source of iron—but as with protein, it is not the only source. Iron in foods comes in two forms: heme and nonheme. Heme iron is more easily absorbable by your body than nonheme iron. Heme iron is found in beef, yes, but it is also found in poultry and fish. Nonheme iron is found in both animal-based foods and plant foods. You can increase the amount of iron (heme and nonheme) your body can absorb if you eat foods that are rich in vitamin C at the same time you eat foods that contain iron. Sources of vitamin C include citrus fruits, tomatoes, strawberries, mangos, papayas, peppers, potatoes, and cabbage.

The RDA for iron for the average adult male is 10 milligrams. For the average adult female, the RDA is 12 milligrams. For women over the age of 51, the RDA drops slightly to 10 milligrams. Pregnant women need more than twice as much iron (to support the growing fetus)—30 milligrams per day. And lactating women need 15 milligrams per day. If you eat a well-balanced diet, you'll have no problem meeting the RDA for iron. Pregnant women are commonly advised by their doctors to take an iron supplement to ensure enough iron is present to support the pregnancy.

Here are some common foods that contain iron:

- Steamed clams (3 ounces)—24 milligrams iron
- Tofu, raw, firm (½ cup)—14 milligrams iron

- Red kidney beans (1 cup)—5 milligrams iron
- Tenderloin steak, choice (3½ ounces broiled)—4 milligrams iron
- Artichoke (1 medium boiled)—4 milligrams iron
- Spinach (½ cup boiled)—3 milligrams iron
- Dried almonds (1 ounce or 24 nuts)—1 milligram iron
- Raisins (¼ cup)—1 milligram iron

For decades, doctors have advised women who were menstruating to eat beef as means of increasing the amount of iron in their diets and thus in their bodies. (Blood loss reduces the amount of iron in the body.) This probably did the trick for most women who had iron-poor blood—the common term for anemia. But it probably also gave women far more fat, especially saturated fat, and calories than they needed. By eating a variety of lower-saturated-fat, iron-based foods, you can take in enough dietary iron without indulging in beef.

IRON SUPPLEMENTS AND IRON POISONING

Healthy adults can get the amount of iron they need through a balanced diet. While doctors may prescribe iron supplements for specific conditions, iron supplements are not for everyone; you should consult with your doctor if you are thinking about taking them. Recent studies suggest that high levels of iron in the body can possibly increase the risk of some conditions, such as heart disease. Although more research is needed to determine the precise relationship between iron and heart health, medical experts recommend that you take iron supplements only if your doctor prescribes them.

Getting too much iron is very dangerous and can even be fatal. Iron poisoning is more likely to happen if you're taking iron supplements, and it is a particular risk for young children whose bodies have a narrow tolerance. Iron supplement tablets often have a candy-flavored coating and are brightly colored, making them attractive to young children. It doesn't take many tablets to result in a fatal level of iron in a child's body. If you are taking iron supplements, be sure to keep them in a child-resistant container and stored in a cabinet that is out of the reach of children.

THE NO-BEEF WAY TO PROTEIN AND IRON

There are many ways to enjoy a healthy diet and still meet your body's needs for protein and iron—without eating beef. Many plant foods, such as the ones mentioned in this chapter, are good sources for these vital nutrients. Balance is a key factor for a healthy diet. Chapter 8 provides more information about food sources for these and other nutrients. The recipes in Chapters 13 through 16 help you stretch your nutritional tastes to include new foods.

6

Fat and Cholesterol

Fat and cholesterol have been deemed almost as evil villains, robbing us of our health and well-being. With numerous warnings about them, fat and cholesterol are two dietary constituents of beef that we need to address. This chapter helps you learn not only more about beef but also about fat and cholesterol in general.

Fat: The Evil Villain to Completely Avoid?

Reduce, reduce, reduce—*total*, that is, *all* fat. This has been the simplified public policy message of recent decades. Indeed, fat is the most caloric thing we find in food; and, well, a lot of Americans have been getting more than their fair share of calories. Obesity, including obesity in our kids, has been rising and continues to rise at astronomical rates. And the risk of many unhealthy complications—from diabetes to heart disease—increases as body fat (not so much body weight) increases beyond what is considered a desirable range.

But fat in your diet is needed in some degree, just not on a large basis. Fat serves a number of purposes, both in foods and in your body. In foods, fat contributes to the satisfying flavor and aroma. Fat also carries the fat-soluble vitamins as well as essential fatty acids. In your body, fat nourishes your skin and hair, helps keep you warm by insulating your body against cold temperatures, provides a protective layer around your vital organs, is part of the outer lining of each of your cells, and gives you a source of energy (calories) as well as an energy reserve (those beloved fat stores) for times when food is scarce.

ALL FATS ARE NOT (STRUCTURALLY) CREATED EQUAL

"Food" fat in all forms, whether in a stick of butter or a tablespoon of oil, contains basically the same amount of calories—9 calories per gram, or 45 calories per serving.

Although they share similar caloric contents, food fats affect your heart health differently. There are primarily three forms of food fats: saturated, polyunsaturated, and monounsaturated. Trans fat is also found naturally in our foods, but on a relatively small basis. Most of the trans fat in our diet today is artificially produced during food processing. As mentioned in Chapter 3, the names given to the different kinds of food fats have to do with the amount of hydrogen present in their chemical structures. Let's look at the different food fats and how they relate to heart health.

Saturated Fats

Saturated fats are completely "saturated" with hydrogen. Because of this, they remain firm, even at room temperature. Saturated fat has been shown to raise blood cholesterol levels. Sources of this fat include butter, bacon grease, shortening and lard, beef fat, and poultry fat.

Polyunsaturated Fats

Fat that is not completely full of hydrogen is called polyunsaturated. These fats are soft or liquid at room temperature. Polyunsaturated fat has not been shown to affect blood cholesterol levels, one way or another. Sources of polyunsaturated fat include corn oil, safflower oil, and soybean oil.

Monounsaturated Fats

Monounsaturated fat has one place in its chemical structure that is free of hydrogen. Liquid at room temperature, these fats have been shown to improve total blood cholesterol levels by raising the level of high-density lipoproteins in the blood. Sources of monounsaturated fat include olive oil, canola oil, avocados, and nuts (such as almonds, peanuts, and cashews).

Trans Fatty Acids

Trans fatty acids are primarily produced during food processing, which involves adding hydrogen to an otherwise unsaturated oil, such as soybean oil. Watch carefully for the terms *hydrogenated* and *partially hydrogenated* oil, to see whether they appear on food labels; these terms indicate that trans fatty acids are present. Trans fatty acids have been shown to negatively affect blood cholesterol levels as much as does saturated fat.

Cholesterol

Cholesterol is another member of the fat family, and it is present in food and in the human body. Your blood (or serum) cholesterol level is, as the name implies, the amount of cholesterol that is present in your blood. Too much blood cholesterol has been shown to increase the risk of heart disease.

HEALTHY BLOOD CHOLESTEROL LEVELS

The level of cholesterol in your blood is not the same as the level of cholesterol in your diet, and it is the level of cholesterol in your blood that matters more when it comes to your heart health. During routine physical examinations for adults, most health-care providers include a blood test to measure the amount of cholesterol in your blood. Elevated levels can indicate an increased risk for heart disease. Total blood cholesterol is a measure of the different types of cholesterol in your bloodstream. The proportion of each type is what really determines your risk for heart disease. It is important to have annual check-ups with your primary care physician, and be sure to track your cholesterol level. A blood cholesterol panel (series of tests) measures the following:

- **Total cholesterol.** This measures the overall cholesterol in your blood and is not very useful by itself. Health experts consider a total cholesterol level between 200 and 239 milligrams per deciliter of blood (mg/dL) as borderline and a level greater than 240 mg/dL as high risk for heart disease. A desirable total cholesterol level is 160 to 199 mg/dL.
- **High-density lipoproteins (HDL).** This measures the amount of HDL cholesterol in your blood. The *higher* this number, the better. A desirable HDL level is 40 mg/dL or greater.
- **Low-density lipoproteins (LDL).** This measures the level of LDL cholesterol in your blood. The *lower* this number, the better. Doctors like to see an LDL level below 130 mg/dL; an LDL level between 130 and 160 mg/dL is borderline and above 160 mg/dL is high risk for heart disease.
- **Ratio.** The cholesterol ratios indicate the relationships between different lipid levels, such as HDL and LDL or HDL and total cholesterol. Health experts like to see a HDL to total cholesterol ratio below 5; the American Heart Association (AHA) considers 3.5 ideal. If your total cholesterol is 200 and your HDL is 50, then your ratio is 4 (200 divided by 50).

As is the case with most medical tests, it's important for doctors to consider your cholesterol levels in the context of your overall health picture. If you smoke two packs of cigarettes a day, consider french fries your favorite vegetable, and get most of your exercise walking to the refrigerator during commercials, a borderline cholesterol level is probably going to catch your doctor's attention (and result in suggestions to make some lifestyle changes). You have additional risk factors for health problems, such as heart disease, that make your cholesterol levels more significant.

Blood cholesterol levels among Americans remain a significant health concern for medical experts. In 2001, a panel of experts convened by the National Institutes of Health's National Heart, Lung, and

Blood Institute (NHLBI) recommended intensified action by doctors and other health-care professionals to reduce the risk for heart disease by lowering the blood cholesterol levels of their patients. The panel said that 65 million Americans—a third of the adult population—need to make dietary and lifestyle changes to bring their blood cholesterol levels down; they recommended that doctors prescribe lipid-lowering drugs for patients who do not make the changes. The leading lifestyle changes the panel encouraged? Eat less fat, especially the fat primarily found in beef (saturated fat), and get more exercise.

DIET AND BLOOD CHOLESTEROL LEVELS

Now, it seems logical that the amount of cholesterol in your diet would directly affect your blood cholesterol levels. Therefore, reducing dietary cholesterol would be a good way to reduce blood cholesterol. Yes? Well, no—at least not in most people. There are a few individuals who are indeed affected by dietary cholesterol. You'd probably know if you were one of them, because you'd have very high levels of blood cholesterol and your doctor would have told you. These people need to be cautious of the amount of cholesterol they eat. For the majority of us, however, this is not the case.

But the general message from organizations like the AHA is for all of us to limit our dietary cholesterol to no more than 300 milligrams per day (or lower if you have a tough-to-treat high blood cholesterol level; your doctor will let you know if this is the case for you). This is to provide a safety net for those who aren't aware that they are affected by the cholesterol they eat. But it's actually good advice for all of us. Lowering foods that are high in cholesterol usually means we are lowering foods high in saturated fat, generally the real culprit of increasing blood cholesterol levels. Foods high in cholesterol tend to be foods high in saturated fat, such as that juicy prime rib.

Monounsaturated fats, on the other hand, have been shown to be positive influencers of blood cholesterol levels. You may have heard about olive oil (which primarily contains monounsaturated fat) as being healthy for our hearts. Well, give me a salad and let me pour it on! Not so fast—remember, *all* fats are rich sources of calories. So you'll want to use even olive oil in moderation. Yes, we want to have some fat in our diets, and fat is not altogether bad. If we want to keep our hearts healthy, though, the primary source fat in our diets should be monounsaturated fat.

The AHA recommends that barely a third (30 percent) or less of our daily calories should be from fat. (The "less" should not generally go below 15 percent according to the World Health Organization.) If you have severe heart disease, your doctor may recommend that you follow the Ornish plan, under close medical supervision. Established by Dr. Dean Ornish, the plan restricts fat intake to no more than 10 percent of calories per day.

Within the recommended 30 percent or less rule, the majority of the fat in your diet should be in the form of monounsaturated fat (10 to 15 percent), with polyunsaturated fat totaling around 10 percent, and saturated fat restricted to no more than 7 percent of total calories. This means that if your recommended daily calorie intake is 2,000 calories, no more than 600 of those calories should come from fat (about 67 grams), of which no more than 200 calories (about 22 grams) should come from saturated fat. What exactly do these numbers mean? Guidance from a registered dietitian in consultation with your doctor would be helpful in determining the amount of calories and fat you should be consuming.

Following the dietary guidelines we provide in our Beef Buster menu planner will help you get started in establishing a low-fat, healthy way of eating.

The Omega-3 Factor

Researchers first became interested in omega-3 fatty acid (linolenic acid) after noticing that people whose diets included large amounts of fish—such as the native population in Greenland—had much lower rates of heart disease than people who seldom ate fish. A number of studies suggest that omega-3 fatty acids found in certain fish (such as salmon and mackerel), flaxseed, and walnuts appear to be protective against heart disease. Omega-3 fatty acids also seem to be protective against stroke, age-related eye disease, and depression.

The Fat Serving Size Challenge

Because we need some fat in our diet, it's important to be aware of the serving sizes of the fat sources in our diet, or we may consume far too many calories. Even if you eat primarily foods containing heart healthy monounsaturated fats and omega-3 fatty acids, it's still important to be aware of proper serving sizes, or the benefits of eating "good" fat will be canceled by the negative consequence of getting too many calories: obesity.

A serving of "table" fat is fairly straightforward. It means 1 teaspoon of butter, margarine, vegetable oil (such as corn, olive, safflower, soybean, canola, peanut), regular mayonnaise, bacon grease (ew!), and shortening or lard. One serving of fat also equals 2 tablespoons cream (or half-and-half), 1 tablespoon regular cream cheese, 1 tablespoon regular salad dressing, 2 tablespoons of coconut, and 10 large green (stuffed) olives. But where people really get tripped up is with the portion sizes of meats, beef in particular.

The American Dietetic Association recommends that a serving size of meat should be about 3.5 ounces of cooked meat. This is smaller than many of us might think is a standard serving. Exactly how big is this? A 3.5-ounce piece of cooked beef or poultry is about the size and thickness of a deck of cards—just about enough to cover the palm of an average adult woman's hand.

The portions most people eat are significantly larger than the recommended serving size. If your home-cooked hamburger patty overlaps the edge of the standard-size bun (or fits nicely into a king-size roll) and takes a wide bite to eat—it could weigh in at as much as 8 ounces or more. That's more than twice the 3.5-ounce healthful cooked weight target. An 8-ounce steak looks pretty small by restaurant standards; it's not uncommon for restaurants to offer steaks that weigh in at 1 pound or more (though most weights listed in the menu are before cooking, so what comes to your table is generally 20 to 25 percent less). It's these real-life portions that cause people to underestimate the amount of beef—and fat—that they consume.

Another challenge is that most people underestimate how much they eat. Researchers find that, in general, people who are of healthy weight underestimate how much they eat by about 20 percent and people who are overweight underestimate their food intake by about 30 percent. According to U.S. Department of Agriculture surveys, as many as 30 percent of Americans falsely believe their diets contain the right amount of fat, and as many as 42 percent believe their diets are healthier than they actually are.

Making Leaner Choices

Although some cuts of beef can be as lean as some kinds of chicken, beef almost always has more fat (most notably saturated fat) than a comparably sized portion of other meat product. An individual cut of beef can be bumped up to a higher fat level if it has a particularly large fat deposit or down to a lower level if it is very well trimmed (or if you remove the skin from poultry). If you eat the fatty trim on any meat or the skin on any poultry, you're eating nothing but fat!

How you cook meat also affects its fat content. Broiling, grilling, and baking are relatively low-fat cooking methods, because they allow the fat and grease to drain away. Frying and braising the meat in its own juices are higher fat cooking methods. Rinsing ground beef in hot water after cooking can also reduce the amount of fat. See the table for the fat content of some common foods.

FAT CONTENT OF SOME COMMON FOODS

Food	Saturated Fat (grams)	Total Fat (grams)	Calories (grams)
Ground beef, broiled (3.5 ounces)			
Regular	8	21	290
Extra lean	6	16	255
Chicken and turkey, roasted (3.5 ounces)			
Light meat with skin	4	14	240
Light meat without skin	1	5	175
Fish, grilled or steamed (3 ounces)			
Tuna	1	5	155
Halibut	0	3	120
Milk, cow's (1 cup)			
Whole	5	8	150
Low fat (1 percent)	2	3	100
Nonfat (skim)	0	0	90
Table fat (1 tablespoon)			
Lard	5	13	110
Butter	8	13	120
Olive oil	2	14	125

SOURCE: Jean A. Pennington. *Bowes and Church's Food Values of Portions Commonly Used*, 17th ed. (Philadelphia: Lippincott-Raven, 1998).

Striking a Healthy Balance with Fat

Your body needs some fat from your diet. To give it the healthiest supply, choose foods that are high in monounsaturated fats and low in saturated fats. As you reduce or eliminate beef, you will greatly reduce your saturated fat intake. If you enjoy animal protein, make it fish instead of beef—you will not only reduce the amount of saturated fat that you eat but you will also get heart healthy omega-3 fatty acids.

7

Other Meats, Dairy, and Fish Too

You don't have to give up your favorite flavors and dining experiences to cut back on the beef you eat. With a little imagination (and the recipes in Chapters 13 through 16), you'll find that it's easy and fun to explore new ways to enjoy old delights. Chapter 14's A Better Burger features a blend of extra-lean ground beef and ground turkey breast combined with onions, pickles, lettuce, and other delectable ingredients—plus your own special blend of condiments, nonfat, if you desire—for only 300 calories and 10 grams of fat (3 grams saturated). You're allowed that blend of beef and turkey as long as you grind your own beef at home from a piece of red muscle meat. You don't have to completely give up the beef right away! Compare that to the McDonald's Big Mac, which packs 560 calories and 34 grams of fat (11 grams saturated). And the recipes in Chapters 15 and 16 should make you see that beef doesn't have to be included at all for a wonderful, satisfying meal experience.

You might even discover that, without your beef habit to define your options, there are many more choices available to you. They are choices that have always been there, of course—but your focus on beef kept you from seeing them. Expanding your tastes to increase your selections from other foods such as fruits, vegetables, and grains will help you to eat a more balanced diet.

This chapter presents an overview of different kinds of protein-rich foods other than beef. Use this information to broaden your thinking about what you eat, and then try out some of the recipes later in the book. You're on a grand and glorious adventure—take a look and enjoy!

High-Protein, Low-Fat Alternatives to Beef

A single ounce of beef supplies 7 grams of protein—along with 3 to 8 grams of saturated fat, depending on the cut and how it is cooked. But there are plenty of other choices that give you just as much protein per ounce with much less fat. Legumes have virtually no saturated fat, and the omega-3 fatty acids in certain fish have shown to be good for your heart. Here's how other foods with the same amount of protein—7 grams—stack up.

- **High protein, very lean.** Foods that supply 1 gram of fat or less and 35 calories per ounce include skinless white meat poultry, halibut, cod, tuna canned in water, clams, crab, lobster, shrimp, dried beans and peas, lentils, and egg whites.
- **High protein, lean.** Foods that supply 3 grams of fat and 55 calories an ounce include skinless dark meat poultry, fresh ham, cottage cheese, Parmesan cheese, oysters, herring, sardines, salmon, catfish, and tuna packed in oil.
- **High protein, medium fat.** Foods that supply 5 grams of fat and 75 calories an ounce include dark meat poultry with skin, pork top loin, pork cutlet, pork loin chop, fried fish, feta cheese, mozzarella cheese, ricotta cheese, and eggs.

Most beef cuts fall into the high-protein, medium-fat grouping. In the high-protein, high-fat group, you'll find processed meats, sausage, bacon, and hot dogs. They also provide 7 grams of protein per ounce, but they contain the same amount of fat. You are better off getting your protein from lower fat foods.

THE OTHER WHITE, OR RATHER RED, MEAT: PORK

Pork has been widely promoted as the other white meat, a reference more to the color of its flesh when cooked—white—than to its fat content. Technically, pork is a red meat, and generally it is higher in total fat and saturated fat than true white meats such as chicken or turkey. (Of course, your choice of cut and preparation style affects leanness.) A 3.5-ounce broiled serving of lean pork center loin, for example, contains 8 grams of fat (3 grams saturated) and 200 calories. This is fairly comparable to many medium-fat cuts of beef.

Pork might add variety to your diet, but there are other animal meats that are lower in saturated fat than pork; and ultimately, these should be emphasized more than pork. Increasingly, you'll find ground pork in the freezer case at your local supermarket. Ground turkey or chicken remains the lower-fat choice. Always cook pork until the juices run clear; pork should reach an internal temperature of 170°F to kill any pathogens that might be present.

Ham is another form of pork. A 3.5-ounce center slice of regular ham contains about 226 calories and 15 grams of fat (5 grams saturated). But the same slice of lean ham contains about 136 calories and 5 grams of total fat (1.6 grams saturated). Lean ham is a good low-fat substitute for bacon (high in fat) in many recipes. Ham comes fresh (uncooked) or cured (ready to eat). Cook fresh ham to an internal temperature of 160°F. Health experts also recommend that you heat precooked ham to an internal temperature of 140°F before eating, just to be sure there are no pathogens lingering to make you ill.

One nutritional drawback to ham, however lean, is its high salt content. A 1-ounce slice of ham contains about 340 milligrams of sodium. By comparison, a 1-ounce serving of pork loin has just 25 milligrams of sodium. Health experts generally recommend that your diet contain no more than 2,400 milligrams of sodium (in all forms) daily. Salt—technically known as sodium—has been a popular preservative since ancient times. Before the advent of refrigeration and canning, people commonly preserved meats by surrounding them with salt, and today's cured meats typically are high in sodium, too. These meats include bacon (regardless of meat source), corned beef, beef jerky, and ready-to-eat sausages such as pepperoni and salami. Many processed meats and hot dogs (beef, turkey, pork, or a combination) also contain high levels of sodium.

Doctors often recommend that people with hypertension cut back on the sodium they consume, both as added salt and in processed foods. The average American consumes 4,000 milligrams or more of sodium a day, an amount well beyond that which is necessary to meet the body's needs. Your body uses sodium to maintain its fluid balance, transmit signals between nerve cells, and conduct electrical impulses through your heart.

ALSO FROM THE COW: DAIRY PRODUCTS

Beef isn't the only food that comes from a cow. Dairy products such as milk, cheese, yogurt, sour cream, and cottage cheese are sources of protein, calcium, vitamin D, and other substances your body needs. Because they are animal-based, dairy products also contain saturated fats. Luckily, most dairy products are available in low-fat or nonfat forms, which taste just as good as the regular varieties. These are easy substitutions to make, especially when using dairy products such as sour cream or milk in recipes. If you choose to adopt a vegetarian diet that doesn't include dairy foods, you can use calcium-fortified soy-based milk, cheese, and yogurt instead. Calcium is crucial for bone health; the Beef Busters nutrition plan recommends getting at least two sources of low-fat or nonfat dairy products (or calcium-rich dairy alternatives) a day to ensure adequate calcium intake.

What is the risk of consuming dairy products with regard to mad cow disease? According to the Centers for Disease Control and Prevention (CDC) European traveler's guidelines, milk and milk products as of the time of this book's first printing are not thought to present a risk for passing on the bovine spongiform encephalopathy (BSE) agent.

CHICKEN AND EGGS

Chicken is what most people think of when they think in terms of white meat. In the United States, chicken is easily available. It is also versatile, lending itself to preparation as a stand-alone meat—broiled, fried, grilled, barbecued, or baked—or mixed in recipes ranging from fajitas to stir-fries. White meat chicken—chicken breast—is a relatively lean source of protein (provided you trim all visible forms of fat and remove the skin—which contains a high amount of fat—before eating). Chicken, of course, is not all white meat. Dark meat chicken, such as thighs and legs, is higher in fat (total and saturated) than white meat.

Be sure to trim any visible fat from chicken before cooking. Even chicken breasts often have strips of fat. Aside from the fat itself, the part of the chicken with the highest fat content is the skin. Some people like to cook chicken with the skin on, and then remove the skin before serving or eating. While this keeps the chicken moist, it also adds some fat content. Try cooking chicken in the microwave for juicy, tender meat (but be sure not to overcook, which will make for tough, rubbery meat). Always cook chicken until the juices run clear; chicken should reach an internal temperature of 170°F. This is essential to kill any bacteria that might be present, thus avoiding food-borne illness.

Ground chicken is gaining popularity. Lower in saturated fat and versatile, it is a healthy alternative to ground beef. Always cook ground chicken, like other ground meats, thoroughly.

Do you love the taste and crispy texture of fried chicken? You don't have to give it up to trim the fat from this American favorite. You can coat a skinless chicken breast with a light breading of crushed cracker crumbs (or flaky ready-to-eat cereal), spray with a no-fat vegetable spray and bake in the oven. This is just one of many ways to keep the flavors you crave, while still reducing your saturated (and total) fat intake.

Eggs have gotten a bad rap in recent for their high cholesterol levels. But as noted in Chapter 6, dietary cholesterol doesn't affect blood cholesterol levels in the majority of people. Still, the American Heart Association (AHA) recommends limiting eggs to 4 or less per week. Eggs are high in cholesterol—a large egg contains about 215 milligrams of it, all in the yolk. The AHA also recommends keeping daily cholesterol intakes to 300 milligrams or less. Egg whites are considered to be a "free" food, not limited by cholesterol-reducing recommendations. Egg whites are also very low in calories, with just 20 (a whole egg contains about 80 calories—still low when you take into account how much protein you're getting in an egg), and are fat free. So, indulge in egg whites, if you want, and use in as many recipes as desired! Two egg whites can be substituted for one whole egg in a recipe.

Eggs are also high in protein—one egg contains about 6 grams. And they provide vitamin A, vitamin D, vitamin B_{12}, and iron. Most of these nutrients are found in the yolk. If an egg is cracked when you take it out of the carton, throw it away. Cracked eggs can be contaminated with dangerous *Salmonella* bacteria. Cook eggs until neither the white nor the yolk is runny.

NOT JUST FOR THANKSGIVING: TURKEY

It's turkey that might rightfully be called the other white meat. Most Americans think of turkey only in November. But turkey is a relatively inexpensive, excellent lean meat you can enjoy year-round. Sliced skinless, white meat turkey breast can have as little as 1 gram of saturated fat per 3.5-ounce cooked serving (3.2 grams of total fat, and only 157 calories)—great between two slices of whole grain bread. Turkey is also great in casseroles and soups. Turkey must be cooked to well done—until the juices run clear and the internal temperature reaches 180°F for a whole turkey. Use cooked turkey in soups, casseroles, and other dishes.

Some nutrition resources recommend substituting ground turkey for ground beef in recipes. If you choose to do this, make certain that the product you buy contains only ground turkey. Check the label, ask your butcher, or contact the manufacturer directly. Some commercially packaged ground turkey (and ground chicken, which isn't quite as common) also includes beef by-products that are ground into the mixture to add texture and flavor.

The CDC has warned travelers against eating ground beef when in Europe and other areas where mad cow disease has been detected in cattle. In the same light, we caution you to look for other alternatives to ground meat, especially if you aren't sure of the origin of the meat. There are a number of soy-based products that simulate ground meat or can add a similar texture and flavor to many dishes.

Ground meats and sausages that contain beef by-products carry an increased risk for contamination with spinal cord and organ tissues, which are the parts of the cow where researchers believe the infectious agent that causes mad cow disease concentrates. Many sausage products, particularly kielbasa, typically contain a blend of meats. Turkey sausage and turkey kielbasa are okay to include in your recipes if you can verify that they contain absolutely no beef or beef by-products (including the casings, which are sometimes made from pork instead of beef). Some companies that market organic foods offer turkey kielbasa that is beef-free. If you have any doubts about whether a sausage product contains beef, your safest choice in protecting against the threat of mad cow disease is to make a different selection.

FROM THE WATER: FISH

Fish, both fin and shell, are low in low-saturated fat and high in protein. Some fish are high in omega-3 fatty acids—the polyunsaturated "good" fats. Studies also suggest that omega-3 fatty acids help keep fatty deposits from collecting inside artery walls and keep clots from forming that could break away to cause a heart attack or stroke. Some experts recommend that you eat fish high in omega-3 fatty acids at least twice a week to enjoy this health benefit. Omega-3 fatty acids are highest among cold-water fin fish such as salmon, albacore tuna, mackerel, sardines, herring, and deep lake trout. Shellfish also contain omega-3 fatty acids, though not in as high quantities as these fin fish. Always cook fish until the flesh is opaque and flakes easily. Poaching and steaming are cooking methods that help fish stay moist.

There has been some confusion about whether shrimp is good for you. While shrimp is high in dietary cholesterol—150 milligrams in a 3.5-ounce serving—it is also low in fat, having just 2 grams. This compares to a same-size serving of regular ground beef which has 110 milligrams of cholesterol and 20 grams of fat. For healthy adults with no existing heart disease and no additional risk factors for heart disease, the cholesterol in shrimp and other shellfish is inconsequential compared to the nutritional benefits they provide.

OH, THE JOY AND BENEFITS OF BEANS

Beans, as well as peas and lentils, are a wonderfully low-calorie, economical alternative to beef. No need to worry about *Escherichia coli,* *Salmonella,* or even mad cow disease with these protein-rich plant foods! Full of vitamins, minerals, fiber, and phytochemicals, they are a chronic-disease-fighting food group that should be included in your weekly (if not daily!) eating plan. (See Chapter 9 for more on phytochemicals.)

Toss them in a salad, drop in a soup, add to spaghetti sauce, or top your pizza: Beans add flavor, texture, and a fulfilling "umph" to a variety of foods. Give them (fully cooked) to your toddler to nibble on—beans are wonderfully textured foods for little ones. Check out some of the recipes in Chapters 13 through 16, to see how you can easily incorporate beans and lentils into your diet.

Worried about getting intestinal gas with beans? Adding large amounts of fiber-rich foods of any kind poses the risk of getting some intestinal discomfort. The key is to start out small with just a few beans at a time—perhaps you could add some to your salad—and then gradually increase your intake. Thoroughly rinse beans before eating, whether you are eating them from a can or from your own pot, to rinse away some of the carbohydrates that may be giving you discomfort. Several commercial products are available that you can buy to help you digest beans.

Low-Fat Cooking Methods

How you fix the foods you eat has a great deal to do with their fat content. A 5-ounce, deep-fried, breaded chicken breast from KFC brings 400 calories and 24 grams of fat (6 grams saturated) to the table. A similarly sized portion of oven-fried skinless chicken breast, coated with nonfat cooking spray to provide crispness, has about 140 calories and 3 grams of fat (1 gram saturated).

Cooking methods that allow fat to drain away from food include steaming, broiling, roasting, baking, and grilling. When grilling, try not to char foods. Some studies link eating charred meats with an increased risk for certain cancers, such as colon cancer. Frying adds fat to any food. Braising, stewing, and poaching do not let the fat drain away, and thus can be high in fat (unless you skim all the fat from the broth). Low-fat cooking methods, safely used, are recommended for optimal health. Drain that fat away!

8

A Healthy Weight and a Balanced Diet

Evidence linking eating habits, weight, and health continues to mount. In fact, health experts worry that contemporary Westerners are eating their way to early graves. A Rand Corporation study reported in 2001 found that one in five Americans weighs more than is healthy—36 percent of Americans are overweight, and 23 percent are obese. The study found that people who are obese have twice as many chronic health problems as people who are of healthy weight, more than people who smoke or drink to excess.

Researchers in other countries are reaching similar findings. At the 11th European Conference on Obesity, held in 2001, researchers reported that more than 90 percent of adults with type 2 diabetes are overweight or obese. Yet a weight loss of just 5 to 10 percent could be enough to prevent as many as 57 percent of these cases, the researchers said. Overweight and obesity are increasing throughout Europe, affecting an average of 20 to 30 percent of Europeans.

As Western eating habits spread throughout the world, so too do the problems associated with them. Health officials from China, for example, are concerned about rising overweight and obesity in their country, which they attribute to rapidly changing eating habits as red meat gains prominence in the Chinese diet. While the overall obesity rate remains relatively low in China—5 percent—it doubled between 1982 and 1992 and appears to be on track for even more rapid growth over the next decade. In the country's more developed areas, as many as 30 percent of people are overweight, a proportion approaching that of Europe and the United States.

The Weight Crisis

Why worry so much about weight? After all, isn't the obsession with thinness a phenomenon of modern times? Statues and paintings from earlier centuries clearly portray bodies considerably more bountiful than the bone-thin models that appear in photographs in today's magazines. But let's not confuse fad and fashion with health.

According to the U.S. Department of Agriculture (USDA), 90 percent of Americans fail to follow dietary guidelines for nutritious eating. One consequence is a rise in the number of people who are overweight or obese. Another is an increase in lifestyle-related health problems such as heart disease and some forms of cancer. (See Chapter 4 for more on cancer.) Why have Americans eaten themselves into record weights? While researchers don't know for sure, there seem to be two key reasons: one rooted in history and one a function of modern times.

Eating has been a sign of social status from the beginning of recorded history. The ability to eat well—and show it—has long been perceived as a reflection of prosperity. Public presentations of this prosperity include bacchanalian delights such as dining out and hosting or attending events ranging from barbecues to lavish dinner parties. Throughout much of history, corpulence has been an individual's personal presentation of prosperity: A plump body shows everyone who sees it that it receives more than adequate nourishment. Being able to build a comfortable cushion of body fat meant that a person ate not only for sustenance but also for pleasure—and often ate expensive and fancy foods that only the rich could afford.

In the past, when few people lived to age 50, there was little reason to be concerned about the cumulative consequences of an excessive lifestyle. An American born in 1900 had a life expectancy of just 47 years. A person born in the United States today can expect to live to age

80 or beyond—almost twice as long. Advances in living conditions and medical technology get most of the credit. We have eliminated many of the diseases that caused death a century ago and are now reducing the consequences of diseases that cause death today.

Now fast-forward to the present. How you live your life makes a difference in how long you will live. If you want to be around for the next 20, 30, 40, or more years, you need to take care of yourself. Eating well is no longer about eating as much as you can afford. Eating well is making food choices that support your body's health. The problem is, many people believe they are eating well, when in fact they are just eating a lot. Studies show that people underestimate the quantity of food they eat each day by as much as a third and that people don't have a good sense of what kinds of foods they eat. We tend to think we eat healthier than we do; most Westerners eat too many foods filled with fats and sugars (meats, dairy, desserts) and too few foods filled with valuable nutrients (fruits, vegetables, whole grains).

What Is a Healthy Weight?

Many different weight charts have been developed over the years to categorize different body weight ranges for different heights. These charts often disagreed with each other. To avoid confusion, a system of measurement called the body mass index (BMI) became the standard weight assessment tool among health-care professionals in the 1990s. The BMI establishes numeric ranges, based on height and weight figures, that correlate to health risks. As your BMI increases, so do your risks for health problems such as diabetes and heart disease. These are the basic BMI ranges:

- BMI 18 to 24.9—ideal for health
- BMI 25 to 29.9—overweight; increased health risk
- BMI 30 or higher—obese; significant health risk

Your BMI is your weight in kilograms divided by your height in meters squared [weight (kg) ÷ height squared (m²)]. You may find it easier to calculate your BMI according to the guidelines provided by the National Institutes for Health:

1. Weigh yourself with no clothes on.
2. Multiply your weight in pounds by 704.5. (Note: the American Dietetic Association, among others, use 700; the difference is inconsequential.)
3. Measure your height with no shoes on.
4. Divide the number you got in step 2 by your height in inches.
5. Divide the number you got in step 4 by your height in inches.

For example, let's suppose you are 5 feet, 8 inches tall and weigh 180 pounds.

1. Weight in pounds: 180.
2. Weight times 704.5: 180 × 704.5 = 126,810.
3. Height in inches: 68.
4. The number from step 2 divided by height: 126,810 ÷ 68 = 1,864.85.
5. The number from step 4 divided by height: 1,864.85 ÷ 68 = 27.4.

In this case, your BMI is 27.4, well into the range of overweight. Now let's say you are 5 feet, 4 inches tall and weigh 115 pounds. Here's your BMI: 115 × 704.5 = 81,017.5; 81,017.5 ÷ 64 = 1,265.9; 1,265.9 ÷ 64 = 19.8. A BMI of 19.8 is in the range of healthy. And if you are 5 feet, 10 inches tall and weigh 225 pounds, your BMI is 32.3, which is in the obesity range. Go ahead, follow these examples and can calculate your own BMI.

The National Institutes of Health and other health experts define overweight as weighing more than a determined standard. Obesity, on the other hand, is the situation of having a high proportion of body fat. People who are obese are also overweight, although people who are overweight can have a healthy body fat percentage. One criticism of the BMI is that it doesn't take into account that muscle tissue weighs more than fat tissue. Correspondingly, someone who is very active physically and has a high level of muscle mass weighs more than someone whose lifestyle involves little movement.

It is possible for your BMI to identify you as overweight when in fact your weight is healthy for your lifestyle. When this is the case, doctors recommend one of several tests to determine your percentage of body fat. One of the simplest is to measure your waist (at your true waist, midway between your hip bones and your belly button). If this measurement is over 35 inches for women or 40 inches for men, your higher BMI is *not* the result of bulked up muscle.

Researchers have established a particular correlation between weight that accumulates around your midsection and an increased risk for heart disease. This is often called the "apple" pattern of weight distribution. People who tend to accumulate weight through the hips and thighs instead have a "pear" pattern, which is not associated so closely with heart disease. However, most health experts believe that excess weight, no matter how you carry it on your body, contributes to a variety of adverse health conditions over time.

The Balance of Healthy Weight

In one respect, body weight is a simple matter of balance. If you eat more calories than your body needs, you gain weight. If you eat fewer calories, or increase your activity level to use more calories, you lose weight. The challenge is to know what balance is right for *you*. While there are general guidelines for typical calorie needs, your personal needs depend on three key factors:

Age. With increasing age comes diminishing muscle tissue. The typical adult loses 2 percent of muscle mass every decade of adulthood, which the body replaces with fat tissue. Muscle is "active" tissue. It burns calories. Body fat is "dead weight." It isn't active, it isn't producing oxygen, and it isn't burning calories. So having less muscle tissue means you don't need as many calories. By age 50, you might need 150 fewer calories a day than required when you were 20 or 25 years old. (Exciting research is under way, however, showing that even elderly people can gain, or regain, lost muscle mass through supervised weight training. Ask your doctor for more information.)

Gender. Men's bodies typically have less body fat than women's bodies. So in general, a man can consume more calories without weight gain than a woman can consume without weight gain.

Activity level. The more active you are, the more calories your body needs and uses. The rate at which your body burns calories goes up during exercise, and continues at an elevated level for some time after exercise. As well, exercise helps you gain muscle mass—and muscle burns more calories.

A diet high in beef is often a diet that lacks balance—nutritionally as well as in terms of calories. And beef can be high in fat and, therefore, calories. Also, beef-dominated diets are most likely lacking in beneficial plant foods, leaving your body shortchanged when it comes to vital nutrients.

Although your body might view the foods you eat in terms of the elemental nutrients they provide, your mind probably thinks in terms of calories. A calorie is a unit of measure. From a nutritionist's perspective, calories measure the energy values of foods and activities. (A chemist defines a calorie as the amount of heat required to cause the temperature of 1 gram of water to rise 1°C.) Technically, these are kilocalories—1,000 calories—or Calories with a big C (the chemist's calorie gets a small c). But the line has blurred between the technically correct and casual use, and most often when you see the word *calorie* with a small c it refers to food and activity energy.

While size might not matter when it comes to the c, it can make a great deal of difference when it comes to the calories' source and, more important, serving size. Gram for gram, fat has more than twice as many calories as protein or carbohydrate. In practical terms, this means that 1 gram of protein or 1 gram of carbohydrate contains energy equal to 4 calories, whereas 1 gram of fat contains 9 calories.

Your body requires a certain level of energy to maintain its functions. A moderately active female adult might use 2,200 calories in 24 hours, and a moderately active male adult may use 2,400. Balance among the energy elements you take in—food—is essential for your body's efficient and effective operations. Most health organizations, including the American Dietetic Association, recommend a diet that gets 55 to 60 percent of its calories from carbohydrates, 10 to 12 percent from protein, and 30 percent or less from fats.

To help achieve these percentage guidelines, the USDA recommends the following distribution of food groups. Of course, consultation with a registered dietitian allows you to determine your individual caloric and nutrient needs.

- Bread, cereal, rice, and pasta group—6 to 11 servings each day
- Vegetable group—3 to 5 servings each day
- Fruit group—2 to 4 servings each day
- Milk, yogurt, and cheese group—2 to 3 servings each day
- Meat, poultry, fish, dry beans, eggs, and nuts group—2 to 3 servings each day
- Fats, oils, and sweets—use sparingly

The Beef Buster menu planner in Chapter 12 fine-tunes these general recommendations to provide more guidelines for incorporating foods that have been shown to promote health and fight chronic disease, such as soy, giving you a practical tool for achieving a beef-free, low-fat, healthy way of eating.

Achieving a Healthy Weight

The American Dietetic Association recommends a general guideline it calls the "Rule of Ten" for approximating your body's basic metabolic caloric needs. Your basic metabolic needs are the amount of calories

Food Guide Pyramid

A Guide to Daily Food Choices

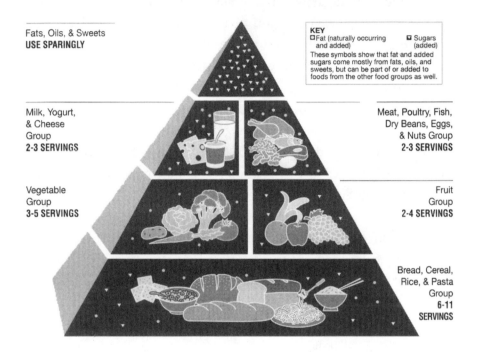

Fats, Oils, & Sweets
USE SPARINGLY

KEY
□ Fat (naturally occurring
and added)
▨ Sugars
(added)
These symbols show that fat and added
sugars come mostly from fats, oils, and
sweets, but can be part of or added to
foods from the other food groups as well.

Milk, Yogurt,
& Cheese
Group
2-3 SERVINGS

Meat, Poultry, Fish,
Dry Beans, Eggs,
& Nuts Group
2-3 SERVINGS

Vegetable
Group
3-5 SERVINGS

Fruit
Group
2-4 SERVINGS

Bread, Cereal,
Rice, & Pasta
Group
**6-11
SERVINGS**

your body needs for general metabolic functions, such as digestion. For every pound of body weight, figure that your body needs at least 10 calories to meet its basic needs for living. If you weigh, say, 150 pounds then you would need about 1,500 calories a day to cover your basic metabolic caloric needs.

To determine your total caloric needs, you will need to figure in the amount of activity you do in a day beyond just breathing, eating, and sleeping. To calculate your total caloric needs, use this quick method. Take your basic metabolic caloric needs, as determined by the "Rule of Ten" formula, and then multiply this number by .60 (it is estimated that your basic metabolic needs are 60 percent of your total caloric needs). Add this number to your basic metabolic caloric number and this gives you an approximation of your total caloric needs to maintain your previous weight.

For example, for the 150-pound person, who needs about 1,500 calories for basic metabolic needs: Multiply 1500 by .60. The result is 900. Add 900 to 1,500 to get 2,400 total calories needed daily for healthy weight maintenance. Of course, these calculations are for general guidelines only. The formula doesn't take into account differences in gender, age, or genetics. To determine your true total caloric needs, it is best for you to consult a registered dietitian who can give you more personalized guidelines.

If you need to lose pounds to achieve a healthy weight, then it is generally recommended that you do not cut your daily calories below your estimated basic metabolic caloric needs. The best way to lose weight is to increase your activity beyond the total amount of calories you consume. In general, a reduction of about 500 calories a day is needed for a safe weight loss, which is ideally no more than 0.5 to 1 pound reduction per week. Studies have shown that this kind of steady weight loss is healthier for your body and more likely to be permanent. You can cut out those 500 calories by limiting what you eat (while maintaining a balanced diet), increasing your activity level (as safely determined by your fitness ability), or as health experts recommend, a combination of both.

If you need to gain weight, then try to increase your caloric intake by 500 calories with nutritionally dense foods for a 0.5 to 1 pound weight gain per week. Again, consultation with a registered dietitian or other qualified health professional is recommended to ensure a safe and effective weight loss or weight gain regime that is tailored specifically for you.

A healthy weight loss, weight gain, or a weight maintenance diet should be well balanced and feature foods that are nutritionally dense, such as whole grains, vegetables, fruits, and legumes. Instead of solely counting calories when you are trying to lose, gain, or maintain weight, you should instead focus on the types of foods you are eating. Keep an eye out for foods that are high in fat and low in nutrients, such as pastries, and use them only in moderation. Most of the time, when you reduce the amount of fatty foods you eat, you also reduce the calories you consume. If you are trying to lose weight or maintain weight, be aware that this is not always the case with some reduced fat or fat-free products, which can contain as many calories (or more!) than the original food item. So, read and compare labels. If you are trying to gain weight, focus on eating ample amounts of foods that are high in monounsaturated fats, such as many nuts and seeds.

Cutting back on food high in saturated fat, such as beef, is not only beneficial in keeping your caloric intake in check, but may help to reduce your risk of heart disease. The Beef Buster meal planner is a well-balanced way of eating, featuring foods that are low in saturated fat, high in nutrients, and that are great tasting. You may find that by following the Beef Buster guidelines, you will lose, maintain, or gain weight without even feeling as if you were dieting.

The Importance of Physical Activity

We won't call it exercise, because that sounds like work. But *physical activity* is what keeps your body moving, and that's as essential as your diet for good health and long life. Activity increases your metabolism, which means your body needs more energy so uses more calories. Health experts recommend a minimum of 30 minutes of activity a day, at least three or four days a week. For optimum health, go for 60 minutes a day five days a week, blending aerobic and other exercise such as weightlifting or resistance training (men and women alike benefit).

Here are some easy ways to make your lifestyle more active:

- Walk. Park your car at the back of the lot instead of in the spot closest to the door. Go around the block at lunchtime or in the evening before dinner. Take the dog or the kids and enjoy some quality time together.
- Take the stairs instead of the elevator or escalator.
- Ride a bicycle or walk to work instead of driving.

- Get up and move around, even just to walk circles around your desk, for a few minutes every hour. While you're sitting at your desk, fidget—jiggle your feet, tap your fingers, shift around in your seat.
- Make a list of the activities you enjoyed when you were a kid. What keeps you from doing them now? Pick one, and do it!
- If you tend to eat (or overeat) when you feel stressed, try indulging in a favorite activity instead of reaching for a high-fat bag of chips or a second serving of roast beef.

You don't have to do your 30 minutes all at once. Take a 10-minute walk at lunch, and then spend another 10 minutes walking the dog or washing the car or doing yard work when you get home. Shoot 10 minutes' worth of hoops with your kids after dinner or take another walk. Activity is activity, and it all adds up. One bonus that comes with splitting up your activity time is that you tend to spend more time being active: 10 minutes really isn't very long, and when the weather's nice it's easy to let that short lunch walk stretch into 15 or 20 minutes.

The False Achievements of Fad Diets

Just about every consumer magazine you pick up has an article about fast and easy ways to lose weight. Any diet that promises a magical solution to a blissful existence by completely eliminating particular food groups should be viewed with caution. "Fast and easy" weight loss means one thing: greatly reducing caloric intake. Any fad diet that severely restricts calories, or advocates one food group at the expense of others, sets up the potential for a variety of health problems.

Your body needs a certain level of calories, particularly in the form of carbohydrates (although protein and fat are important as well), to function adequately. If your diet doesn't meet your body's calorie needs, then your body is forced to turn on itself, switching into starvation mode.

Remember the discussion in Chapter 3 of how carbohydrates are the body's preferred source of energy to fuel its bodily functions? Well, if you severely restrict calories and your diet does not contain enough carbohydrates, then your body looks to your carbohydrate reserves— your glycogen stores (found in the liver and muscle tissue). Ultimately, your body may turn to your lean tissue (such as the tissue in your skeletal muscles, heart, and lungs) to get the protein that will be converted to glucose. If you continue to eat too few or no calories for more than a few days, your body taps into your fat reserves to produce an alternative source of energy for your body. Fat cannot be converted to glucose. What are produced instead are ketone bodies, and your body is therefore fueled in "ketosis" mode.

Advocates of high-protein diets, which typically promote high beef consumption, herald ketosis as a signal that your body is burning fat and you are losing weight. Although being in ketosis involves a reduction of insulin released in your body, which allows you to dip into your fat stores for fuel, it really isn't the ideal way to lose body fat. Ketosis is a process designed to protect your body from the ravages of starvation. It can allow an otherwise healthy person to live six to eight weeks without food. This doesn't mean you should try it.

Ketosis can lead to all sorts of unwanted side effects—from a loss of body water, sodium, and potassium to irregular heartbeats and to gout (if your uric acid level becomes too high). The arguments for the benefits of living in ketosis seem small. Also, when running on an alternative energy source (not glucose), you can feel lightheaded, tired, and have no endurance. Your brain tires, too, making it difficult for you to think clearly, focus, or concentrate. In our opinion, this is not a good way to lose weight, and certainly does nothing to support your overall health and well-being.

If a high-protein diet has you eating lots of beef as a source of protein, shouldn't the fat that you're also getting give your body the calories you need? Not in the short term. Remember, dietary fat is an *indirect* energy source. While it's easy enough for your body to convert excess dietary fat into body fat, the process to convert body fat into usable energy is complex and time-consuming. So excess protein and fat from the beef goes to feed your fat stores, not your body's immediate energy needs.

You might feel fine on such a diet or on a diet that severely restricts your calorie intake—for a while. About half of your nerve and brain cells can draw enough energy from ketone bodies to fuel their functions, just as your car's engine can run even if gasoline doesn't make it to all of the cylinders. But remember that your car won't run well this way; it'll sputter and balk; and so your brain and other body parts won't run well either when they receive just half the fuel they need.

No matter how much you like a particular food, you are going to get tired of it if you eat it all the time. People who lose weight on fad diets tend not only to regain the lost weight when they stop following the diet but, in fact, to gain back even more weight because the body wants to protect itself from, and get ready to withstand, any similar starvation situation in the future. This is one of the negative consequences of what's known as "yo-yo dieting" or diet cycling—going on and off restrictive diets will cause weight to go down, then up—down and then up even higher.

Each bout of weight loss typically involves muscle loss, and the corresponding weight gain phase typically adds more body fat. So if a yo-yo dieter gains back all of the weight he or she lost, the weight distribution will most likely be greater in fat than lean muscle tissue. This means the person can be obese even if the scale weight doesn't show it. This is not good for health.

The best way to lose weight is to make simple adjustments in your eating habits and to gradually increase your physical activity. Seem too easy to be true? Really, it's not. Weight loss should not be a rigorous, painful affair of deprivation. Instead, it should come naturally as part of an improved way of living such as the one on which you are embarking as you cut beef from your daily meals. The Beef Buster guidelines will help you make easy, simple, and enjoyable alterations in your diet that not only will help you lose a few unwanted pounds but also will improve your overall health and sense of well-being.

9

Eating Vegetables
without Being a Vegetarian

Vegetables: "Yuck!" For many of today's adults, this refrain lingers from childhood when eating the greens was the only way to get away from the dinner table. (It doesn't have to be this way; Chapter 10 offers suggestions for getting your kids to like, and even prefer, vegetables.) While most people eventually grow up to like at least some vegetables, few eat as many servings as health experts recommend—three to five daily.

Today's vegetables are about as far removed from those indistinguishable canned greens of the past as you can get. With advances in refrigeration techniques and rapid transportation, it's possible to speed vegetables across the continent to arrive in grocery stores and produce markets fresh and crisp—and still nutritious.

Vegetables and other plant-based foods do more for your diet than help you avoid the risk of mad cow disease that may be present in eating red meat. They are storehouses of nutrients. They contain vitamins, minerals, and hundreds (if not thousands) of phytochemicals—substances unique to plants (not found in animal-based foods such as beef and other meats) that your body uses in countless ways. Scientists are only beginning to understand the complex and intertwined roles of phytochemicals in keeping you healthy and in preventing and even fighting disease. Let's look at some key phytochemicals and the vegetables that contain them.

Flavonoids are a large class of phytochemicals that appear to inhibit the onset of cancer and heart disease. **Isoflavones** are a particular type of flavonoids that are found abundantly in soybeans. Isoflavones have shown promise in preventing the formation of breast cancer and prostate cancer.

Carotenoids appear to play a role in enhancing immunity and in preventing the growth of cancer cells. Brightly colored vegetables such as carrots, sweet potatoes, and tomatoes are high in carotenoids. **Lycopenes,** a type of carotenoid, are thought to prevent and fight prostate and breast cancer. Tomatoes are a rich source of lycopenes. Pink-fleshed fruits such as watermelon and pink grapefruit also contain lycopenes.

Cruciferous vegetables such as broccoli, cauliflower, and cabbage contain **sulforaphanes,** one of the most potent anticancer agents known to researchers.

Phytoestrogens are produced in your intestine after the ingestion of other phytochemicals—flavonoids, isoflavones, and lignans. Phytoestrogens are often referred to as plant estrogens, which are chemically similar to but not the same as human estrogens, and are found in soy-based products. In addition to helping prevent breast and prostate cancer, phytoestrogens also seem to provide relief from menopause discomforts for many women.

Lignans, which are converted to phytoestrogens in the intestine, have shown to be powerful antioxidants, as well as cancer fighters. They are found in whole grains, berries, flaxseed, and many vegetables.

Lutein, a powerful antioxidant, has recently received much attention for its ability to protect against age-related macular degeneration, a common cause of blindness in the elderly. Spinach and collard greens are particularly high in lutein.

Nutrients from the Land

Mother Nature has given us a host of plant foods, providing us with ample amounts of vitamins, minerals, phytochemicals, and antioxidants to help keep us healthy and long lived. Although there are many edible plant foods in the sea (which make up wonderful cuisine delicacies such as vegetarian sushi), we will focus on the more wellknown plant foods of the land.

Peaches, apricots, blueberries, strawberries, cherries, apples, bananas, pears, oranges, pineapple, watermelon, dates, raisins—anyone hungry? **Fruit** is nature's candy, and a healthy food group that is hard to dislike. Rich in powerful disease-fighting phytochemicals and fiber, fruits such as oranges and berries give us ample amounts of vitamin C, and some are good sources of minerals like potassium (such as bananas). Indeed, the old saying "an apple a day to keep the doctor away" has some truth to it. The tomato is classed botanically as a fruit, though most people think of it as a vegetable.

Dark green leafy vegetables are sources of carotene (which your body converts to vitamin A), folate, iron, calcium, magnesium, and potassium. Common members of this group of vegetables are broccoli, chard, greens (collard, dandelion, mustard, turnip), kale, romaine lettuce, spinach, and watercress.

Yellow vegetables are great sources of carotene as well as many other vitamins and minerals. Examples of these vegetables are carrots, pumpkin, squash, sweet potatoes, and yams.

Starchy vegetables provide fiber, potassium, and vitamin B_6. Common starchy vegetables are corn, green (sweet) peas, potatoes, rutabaga, and taro root.

Legumes are good sources of protein and contain many vitamins and minerals, such as folate and iron. They also contain a variety of phytochemicals. Beans (black, kidney, lima, mung, navy, soy), chickpeas (garbanzo beans), lentils, and split peas are all legumes.

Grains (in their *whole* form, not refined unless enriched or fortified) provide fiber, along with B vitamins, vitamin E, and iron. We eat most grains in the form of grain products such as cereals and breads. Some common grains are barley, bulgur, couscous, oats, rye, and whole wheat.

Although **nuts and seeds** have often been associated as fatty foods, the fats that they contain are primarily in the heart-healthy form of monounsaturated fat as well as omega-3 fatty acids. They are also good sources of protein and contain many vitamins (such as folate) and minerals (such as iron). Because they contain fat, they also contain a fair amount of calories, so it's best to eat these wonderful nutritious foods in moderation—about 1 ounce per day. Some common nuts and seeds are almonds, Brazil nuts, cashews, chestnuts, filberts (hazelnuts), macadamia, pecans, pistachios, sesame seeds, sunflower seeds, and walnuts. While many people think of peanuts as nuts, they are actually legumes.

What's Best: Fresh, Frozen, or Canned?

Fresh fruits and vegetables generally provide the highest amounts of nutrients and the "fresh is best" rule usually applies to fruits and vegetables. But if the "fresh" produce you see in your grocery store looks tired and pale, or banged up with a lot of cuts and bruises, chances are many of the vitamins and minerals have been lost in the long journey from the field to your grocery store. If this is the case, opt for canned or frozen vegetables, great alternatives to fresh! Some canned and frozen varieties contain as much (if not more!) vitamins and minerals as fresh, unless you picked the fresh produce yourself or it comes from local sources with minimal transit to your place of purchase.

In many geographic regions, winters don't permit growing fresh produce. But canned and frozen fruits and vegetables help get a variety of produce into your diet in the cold months. Remember: A wide variety of fruits and vegetables provides an abundance of different nutrients for optimal health.

Grains: Whole and Refined

Whole grains are an important source of complex carbohydrates and fiber as well as other nutrients. A whole wheat grain contains all the edible parts of the grain, including the germ or seed from which new plants would grow if the grain were planted. The germ of the wheat is nutrient rich, containing many vitamins and minerals, such as cancer- and heart disease-fighting vitamin E and selenium. The outer layer of the wheat grain, called the bran, is also rich in fiber and in many vitamins. In between the germ and the bran is the pulpy, white material called the endosperm, which contains starch and protein; this would help nourish the new plant if it sprouted. Whole wheat flour is ground from the whole seed and contains visible fragments (such as the bran) of the grain's components.

Refined wheat grain, or refined wheat flour, is ground endosperm. It doesn't contain the bran and germ, which houses most of the fiber, vitamins, and minerals. Think white flour, and you've got the picture. Health experts recommend that most of the breads and cereals you eat come from whole grains, to get the full nutritional benefit of the grain. Not all breads and cereals that are brown are made from whole grains, however. Some products contain a blend of whole and refined grains. Food product labels identify whether the product contains whole or refined grain. Most grain products are also fortified with other important nutrients, such as folate, B vitamins, calcium, and iron. (A food is *fortified* when nutrients that it doesn't naturally have are added to it during processing. An *enriched* food contains added nutrients to replace those lost during the manufacturing process.)

The fiber in grains helps food move efficiently through your digestive system. (See Chapter 3 for more on digestion.) Grains contain mostly insoluble fiber, which stays relatively solid in the intestine and absorbs water. This adds bulk to digestive waste, preventing constipation and making it easier for you to pass it, in the form of stools, from your body. Some grain products, such as oats, contain lots of soluble fiber that has been shown to help eliminate excess cholesterol from the body.

The Incredible, Edible Soybean

Soybeans are the only plant-based food that is a complete protein—and few other foods offer as many preparation or nutritional options. You can eat soybeans boiled or roasted or made into a variety of products including soy flour, textured soy protein, tofu, miso, tempeh, and soy milk. The soybean is finally enjoying the culinary status its nutritional content deserves.

The following common soy products offer tasty and convenient alternatives to meat:

- **Textured soy protein.** A versatile product that's available in many forms, from crumbled granules (which work well in soups and dishes such as lasagna and chili) to products that emulate burgers, hot dogs, and even pepperoni.
- **Tofu.** A product with the texture and consistency of cheese, that's available in various firmnesses. Its very mild flavor is often overpowered by the tastes of other foods in the dish. It can be served by itself (grilled or broiled) or added to other ingredients, as in stir-fries; it takes a marinade well.
- **Tempeh.** A fermented mixture of soybeans and grain in the form of a firm cake. Its hearty, nutty flavor holds up well to grilling; it can be added to stews, chili, and casseroles.
- **Miso.** A fermented paste of soybeans with the consistency of creamy peanut butter that works well in dips and spreads, by itself or mixed with other ingredients; it makes a nice soup base.

Soy-based food products provide an added nutritional advantage: isoflavones. Scientists suspect these phytochemicals play a role in preventing and fighting many diseases. The Food and Drug Administration (FDA) has approved the claim that soy protein can reduce your risk of heart disease, and cancer experts credit soy with helping to make your body inhospitable to some forms of cancer, such as cancer of the prostate and of the breast.

The key isoflavones in soy are genestein and daidzein, which some studies have linked to lowered levels of prostate-specific antigen (PSA), an indicator of prostate cancer growth. Scientists believe these particular isoflavones also enhance the body's immune response, although they don't yet understand the mechanisms by which this happens. Soy isoflavones appear to lower the risk of colon cancer as well as prostate cancer.

Soy also contains phytoestrogens—plant forms of estrogen that are chemically similar but weaker than the estrogen that occurs naturally in a woman's body. Although phytoestrogens are not the same as hormone-replacement therapy (HRT), there are studies that demonstrate their ability to control mild to moderate perimenopausal discomforts, such as hot flashes and night sweats. Because more research is needed to more clearly understand how phytoestrogens function in the human body, most medical experts do not recommend that a woman rely on soy estrogens (or any phytoestrogens, regardless of source) as a substitute for traditional HRT; taking soy is not a substitute for HRT.

Soybean and soybean products contain moderate amounts of fat, mostly in the polyunsaturated form. A 3.5-ounce serving of cooked firm tofu, for example, contains 4.5 grams of total fat, but only 0.7 gram of which is saturated fat. Compare this to a 3.5-ounce top sirloin steak, which has about 8 grams of fat, of which 3 grams are saturated fat, and you can see why tofu is the better heart-healthy choice. Some soy products are made into low-fat or nonfat varieties, such as nonfat soy milk. These products retain the benefits of soy (protein and isoflavones) but have fewer calories.

Soy products, especially boiled or roasted soybeans, in quantities larger than the recommended serving size (½ cup for boiled, ⅓ cup for roasted) can be a challenge for your digestive system to handle. The outer skin of the soybean is tough and fibrous; it takes long cooking times to soften it enough to make your digestive system happy. Some people experience unpleasant digestive distress (gas) when they eat soybeans and soybean products, although no more than they might experience from chowing down on a mega-steak whose high-fat, high-protein content also poses a significant digestive challenge.

If you've had bad experiences with soy foods in the past, try them again. This time use smaller quantities and increase gradually. There have been many advances in soy-based products. Some made from textured soy protein imitate the flavors and textures of meat-based favorite foods such as hamburgers and pepperoni.

TRY THE TOFU MARINADE CHALLENGE

Die-hard beef eaters often balk at the thought of replacing their favorite food with something with such a silly-sounding name as tofu. But tofu is one of the most versatile food products available today. It comes in a variety of textures that allow its use in recipes from dips and spreads to chili and casseroles. While certainly you'll notice that tofu isn't steak, it's less likely that you will notice that tofu isn't meat when you use it in dishes such as stir-fries. Because tofu is very mild, it takes on the flavors of the foods with which you cook it. Marinated tofu tastes like the ingredients in the marinade. Try Chapter 15's Pepper Stir-Fry, for example, and see if you (or your family members) can really tell that most of the "meat" is actually marinated tofu.

Make Vegetables the Main Dish

The Western diet centers on meat. Vegetables and grains are considered side dishes. This is not exactly the way your body would like for you to eat! Few Americans eat as much plant foods, such as vegetables, fruits, and grains, as they should. So flip the tables! Make vegetables the main course. (The recipes in Chapters 15 and 16 give you some ideas to start with.) This not only increases the amounts of plant-based foods that you eat but also allows you to cut back on meats in general without feeling hungry at the end of the meal. Serve several vegetables at the same meal—say, white or sweet potatoes along with green beans and squash. The more variety, the better!

Vegetables and Food Safety

Throughout recorded history, there have been great and tragic famines as the result of damage to crops from insects and plant infections caused by fungi, molds, and bacteria. Modern farmers use chemicals to help them grow healthy crops that produce good yields; without them, it would be difficult to meet today's demand for fruits, vegetables, legumes, and grains. Furthermore, chemicals are sometimes added to crop foods after harvest to help preserve them.

Most Western countries strictly regulate chemical use in growing food crops. In the United States, the Environmental Protection Agency (EPA) approves the chemicals, such as pesticides and fertilizers, that farmers can use and establishes the guidelines and limits for using them. Other agencies, including the U.S. Department of Agriculture, the FDA, and the Food Safety Inspection Service, monitor and enforce EPA standards and regulations. The amounts of chemicals farmers can use are very small and do not pose health risks for most people.

Some people attempt to avoid chemical residue by buying organic produce. In the United States, foods sold as organic must meet certain standards that restrict chemical use during growth and processing. This doesn't mean organic farming is chemical-free; it might use natural substances such as sulfur or copper as pesticides and manure for fertilizer. While arguments abound as to whether organically grown produce is better for you than commercially grown produce, there is as yet no scientific evidence to support that there is any appreciable nutritional difference.

As with beef, safe handling procedures can prevent nearly all potential health problems. Always wash vegetables thoroughly with running water (no soap, though, which leaves its own residue). Use a vegetable brush to scrub produce such as carrots and potatoes. Some people peel fruits and vegetables, but this is more likely to deprive you of vital nutrients than protect you from contamination—and if you don't wash items before peeling, you will simply carry any existing contaminants into the produce's flesh. Remove the outer leaves from leafy vegetables such as lettuce and cabbage and be sure to rinse the remaining leaves thoroughly.

Never cut vegetables with utensils or on cutting surfaces that you have used to cut or prepare meat! Doing so will spread any pathogens that might be in the raw or undercooked meat (beef as well as pork, poultry, and game meats in muscle or ground forms) to the vegetables. While cooking to proper temperatures kills most pathogens in or on meat, we often eat vegetables raw or cooked just until tender. A number of recent *Escherichia coli* O157:H7 outbreaks were traced to cross-contamination of fruits resulting from improper handling.

If You Choose a Vegetarian Lifestyle

Of course, you certainly can choose a vegetarian lifestyle if you like. Eliminating meat from your diet helps protect you from food-borne illnesses, and the risk of mad cow disease. Most health experts believe vegetarians can get all the nutrients they need from their diets, just as meat-eaters can, by making sure they eat foods from all food groups. Soybean-based products are an excellent source of complete protein, for example, and can serve as nutritious meat replacements. If you choose to eliminate all dairy foods from your diet, be sure you get enough calcium (and vitamin D) through other sources such as fortified soy-based drinks, breakfast cereals, and orange juice.

10

Busting Your
Family Free

The only thing harder than making changes in your diet is making those changes alone. It's challenging enough to fix beef-free meals for yourself, but it's really difficult to then turn around and fix familiar favorites for others in your household. Rather than getting caught up in a "this is my food, this is your food" dilemma, your entire family can make the transition to healthier—and safer—eating habits. Remember that the best way to avoid the risk of mad cow disease is to avoid red meat altogether. By preparing some of the recipes given in following chapters, you and your family might be pleasantly surprised by the wide array of new colors, textures, and tastes on your plates, as you work toward a shared goal of reducing and, ultimately, eliminating red meat from your family's diet. You might even find it hard to believe that you've been missing out on all those delicious beef-less meals and discover that eating "good" doesn't mean sacrificing really good taste.

What about a reluctant significant other? This is not always easy. After all, part of being an adult is the freedom to make your own choices, whether or not those choices are wise. Your partner might feel betrayed by your decision to change the way you eat, especially if eating out is one of the social activities you enjoy sharing. (More about how to make healthy menu choices later in this chapter.) Or your partner might feel uncomfortable knowing that what you're doing makes good sense, but he or she isn't quite ready to join you in your new lifestyle.

It might take some doing to get your significant other to recognize that today's crisp, fresh veggies are nothing like the canned mush he or she might still associate from childhood. After all, old perceptions die hard. But be patient. Eventually your partner will come to know and love a few vegetables, and then you can gradually introduce others.

While you have to respect your partner's right to make choices that differ from yours, you also have the right to expect that same respect from your partner. It might take some negotiating to figure out how to best handle meals if your significant other is adamantly opposed to cutting beef from the menu. Each person has to find his or her own reasons and motivations to make changes, no matter what those changes are. If you encounter resistance to trimming or eliminating beef from your household meals, we have a few suggestions:

- Set a positive example. Prepare foods and dishes that you enjoy and be sure your pleasure shows (but no gloating!).
- Present the reasons and health benefits for making these changes. If your partner or family isn't ready to take the beef-free plunge all at once, despite the health benefits and the reduced health risks, then practice the fine art of compromise. Agree to the occasional steak on the grill—but draw the line at continuing to eat ground beef that isn't ground at home to avoid contamination, and sausage products that may contain unsavory (and risky) by-products.
- Always prepare enough food to feed all family members. If no one joins you, you can refrigerate or freeze leftovers.
- Look for ways to make family favorites with less or no beef. (The recipes in Chapters 13 through 16 can get you started.) Remember that you can always substitute *something* for the beef in a recipe—consider chicken, fish, beans, and even tofu! Choose what makes sense for the taste and texture of the dish and don't be afraid to experiment.
- Prepare beef-free dishes for your family's meals and fix alterna-

tives only if other family members specifically ask for them. If practical, have them fix their own alternatives.

■ Discourage cheating binges back to beef by having a home-made fast-food night at home, preparing burgers from beef you've ground safely in your own kitchen from a piece of solid red muscle meat, and fries you know won't be dipped in beef fat before frying. Over time, make the switch to beef and turkey blends, and, eventually, to all turkey, or even veggie burgers.

Eventually, even family members who are loudly vocal with their "where's the beef" complaints will be unable to resist sneaking a taste of whatever smells so good cooking on the stove. Kids most likely will get tired of trying to figure out what they want to eat and will start eating what you serve them—and usually a reluctant partner will, too.

Consistency is important. Once you make the decision to reduce or eliminate beef, if you like it, stick with it. If not, keep trying, if reducing beef or eliminating beef is your goal. If you're preparing or going out for a celebratory dinner, don't return to steaks. Instead, pick a favorite recipe from this book and use festive decorations to identify the meal as special. Your taste buds will adjust to a new flavor or texture in about two weeks. Don't confuse them by giving them what they've just gotten used to not having.

CULTIVATE HEALTHY EATING HABITS EARLY

As researchers are learning more about how heart disease starts, they are realizing that it starts much earlier than previously believed. Studies show that lipid buildup in the arteries can begin in children as young as age 4 or 5, if their diets are high in saturated fat. Since we already know that heart disease is the result of the slow accumulation of damage, these findings raise concerns that future generations will begin to show signs of heart disease at younger ages.

Getting your kids off to a healthy start in terms of what and how they eat is a matter of habit. If children are used to reaching for carrots or apples instead of highly processed snack items, such as store-bought chips or cookies, or chips that contain a lot of saturated fat, when they want munchies, they are well on the way to heart healthy eating. The premise that "you don't miss what you don't have" rings especially true in this context—if there are no highly processed, high-fat snacks available, then the kids aren't going to miss them.

Of course, an occasional cookie or serving of chips isn't going to harm a child whose eating habits are otherwise nutritionally sound. But children who grow up reaching for fruits and vegetables for snacks (and who get plenty of exercise, another important health habit) are less likely to be overweight or obese—another concern of health experts and another risk factor for health problems such as heart disease and some forms of cancer.

The most effective way to help your children establish healthy eating habits is to set a good example for them to follow. Keep plenty of fruits and vegetables in the house, and little in the way of highly processed, low nutrient food items, such as chips, cookies, and candy. You can find small bags of cut veggies, such as cauliflower, broccoli, and carrots in the produce section of your local grocery store—ready-to-eat, healthy snacks, very handy! Kids can raid the home fridge for veggies themselves. (Teach your kids to rinse fruits and vegetables thoroughly under cold running water before eating them.) Make vegetables a part of most meals, and serve fruit or fruit-based dishes for dessert. The return on this investment in your child's health will pay off manyfold in the years and decades to come.

Eating Healthy When Eating Out

If your diet has been primarily beef-driven until now, most of your favorite restaurants are likely to be beef-oriented as well. Steak houses and burger joints are the most popular kinds of restaurants in the United States. While some offer menu options to beef dishes, others might offer only token alternatives. Whether you can continue patronizing your old favorites depends on the menu selections. Many people who transition their eating habits away from beef reach a point where they find it unpleasant to be around the smells and sights of beef, as well as other people who are eating it.

If you are concerned about the potential risk for mad cow disease, you'll want to be doubly sure about what you're eating in restaurants, and where it is coming from. Don't assume that a restaurant's offerings are beef-free—many fast-food and other restaurants use beef fat to flavor french fries, or beef broth to flavor sauces. So, just foregoing that steak or burger may not be enough to offer full protection. When in doubt, ask the restaurant manager or chef to confirm that your menu selection is truly beef-free. If you must have beef, choose a solid piece of red muscle meat, a steak, for example, and avoid ordering menu items that contain ground beef or sausage.

Find new favorite cuisines and flavors as an alternative to beef. This will remove any temptation you might feel to indulge for old time's sake and will give you the opportunity to explore many kinds of foods that you never really considered when beef was the mainstay of your diet. Metropolitan areas typically have a diverse selection of restaurants, including many ethnic specialties as well as health-oriented establishments that offer or feature vegetarian dishes. If you've never tried them, you'll be surprised at how good they are. Here are some choices to consider when in different kinds of restaurants. Once again, if you are unsure about the beef content of a menu selection, ask the restaurant manager or chef to confirm whether or not any beef or beef products are included in the recipe.

Chinese cuisine features dishes that contain many delicious beef-free ingredients, such as chicken, seafood, vegetables, and tofu mixed with rice, noodles, or pancake-like bread. Order steamed, roasted, or stir-fried dishes rather than those that are fried (including fried rice) or deep fried.

Many **Greek** dishes feature poultry, fish, and seafood. If choosing stuffed vegetable dishes, avoid those made with ground meat. Try the beef-free shish kebabs, you will be amazed!

Enjoy the pastas and breads that are the mainstay of **Italian** cuisine, but without cream-based sauces, butter, and other spreads. Choose dishes that feature tomato-based sauces and vegetables. Many Italian restaurants offer vegetable lasagna as well as dishes that use chicken instead of sausage or beef.

Japanese cuisine features wonderfully prepared vegetable dishes. Choose chicken and fish over beef and pork. Many dishes include rice or noodles, plain or in low-fat sauces. Sushi is a favorite with those who have acquired a taste for it—delicate pieces of raw fish with rice wrapped in seaweed or ginger. There is always a health risk when you eat uncooked animal-based foods, so eat sushi only from restaurants you know and trust. (If you are pregnant, however, you might want to avoid sushi entirely.)

Middle Eastern cuisine, like other Mediterranean cuisines, such as Greek and Southern Italian, uses little beef and puts the emphasis on grains, legumes, vegetables, nuts, fish, and poultry. Many dishes are naturally nutritious and incredibly delicious.

In **Mexican** restaurants choose dishes that feature grilled chicken or vegetables, salsas, and green chili sauces. Try to choose dishes made with black or red beans instead of refried beans, which are most often cooked in saturated-fat-filled lard. (Ask your waiter whether the refried beans are cooked in lard.) Opt for soft rather than fried tortillas, to help keep your total fat intake low.

Today's **vegetarian** restaurants serve much more than salads and are a non-beef-eater's dream. From sandwiches and soups to main courses, vegetarian dishes feature nutritious and tasty blends of vegetables, grains, legumes, and nuts.

HEALTHY SNACKING

Snacking often gets the bad rap (sharing blame with poor choices at the dinner table) for overweight and obesity. And certainly snacking contributes to burgeoning beltlines, especially in our sedentary times. However, it is not *that* you snack but rather *how* you snack that leads to problems. Many people reach for high-fat chips and cookies when they feel hungry—and sometimes even when they don't but feel the desire to eat something anyway. While just about every workplace has snack and soda machines, few stock apples and juice instead of candy and soft drinks. When you're hungry and away from home, sometimes your only options are snack foods. Still, there are ways to make healthier choices. When the munchies strike, consider these vending-machine options:

Instead of . . .

> Corn chips, potato chips
> Cookies
> Candy bars
> Soft drink

Try . . .

> Pretzels, crackers, popcorn (unbuttered)
> Fruit bars, ginger snaps, vanilla wafers
> Peanuts, raisins (not chocolate-covered!)
> Fruit juice, vegetable juice, bottled water

Better yet, keep your own stock of nutritious snacks. Instant soups, whole wheat crackers, snack packs of raisins and nuts, baked tortilla chips, and unbuttered microwave popcorn. If you have access to a refrigerator, keep a supply of yogurt, fruit, snack-size veggies (cut up cauliflower, broccoli, carrots, and celery), salsa, even potatoes that you can bake in the microwave for a filling and nutritious snack. In fact, snacking can actually be beneficial. Many nutrition experts encourage snacking to avoid the excess hunger at meal times that can lead to overeating. Healthy snacking doesn't make you fat; to the contrary, it can actually help keep you thin!

To Market, to Market

Unless you've been shopping exclusively at a butcher shop, there's no reason for you to change grocery stores. You are not required to shop exclusively at natural foods markets or health food stores; you can find all the ingredients you need for beefless meals at any grocery store. If you're not sure how to buy good produce, ask the produce department manager for suggestions and advice. Enjoy yourself and take a look around. You might be amazed by the variety of plant-based foods and the many interesting colors and shapes. If you see something that intrigues you, buy it! (Check out the recipes in the following chapters for ideas on how to cook many plant-based foods.) Large chain grocery stores often host cooking demonstrations. While these typically feature specific products, it's a good way to learn more about preparing different kinds of foods.

If the store has a bakery, find out what kinds of breads it makes and when they are freshest. And check out the fish counter to see what seafood is available. (But if the fish you look at smells really fishy and unappealing, don't buy it. It might not be the freshest.) There are often recipe cards on display that give you ideas about how to put a new spin on a common product such as cod or salmon. Sometimes fresh chicken breasts are meatier and have less fat on them than frozen chicken breasts. To save time, buy skinless chicken. But if you want to save money, buy chicken with the skin on and remove it yourself before or after cooking.

To buy the healthiest foods and products, learn how to read package labels. In the United States, all packaged foods must contain labels that state the product's complete ingredients and basic nutritional content. Product labels help you get beyond marketing hype to actually compare factors such as fat content. Take *your* typical serving size into consideration. If you know that you always use more salad dressing than the listed serving size, recognize that this affects the amounts of calories, for example, that you get from the product.

If you are concerned about the risks of mad cow disease, beware

some processed foods! Many items you might be accustomed to buying, such as prepared spaghetti sauces, meat sauces, soups, stews, chili,
and other products might contain red meat, ground beef, or beef by-
products. Even foods you might think of as beef-free, such as vegetable
soup, often contain beef broth or other beef-based flavorings. Mad cow
disease has not yet been found in the United States (and, hopefully,
never will be); but, for maximum protection, it is prudent to follow the
Centers for Disease Control and Prevention (CDC) guidelines for travelers to countries where mad cow disease has been found. That means
eliminating red meat from the diet altogether, or choosing solid pieces
of muscle meat instead of ground meat, sausage, and beef by-products
(which have a greater risk of contamination). Avoid processed foods
that contain beef or beef by-products.

Keep Moving

Without question, dropping the beef in your diet may likely make a
difference in your health. But diet is only half of the equation. A
healthy lifestyle—one that strives to preserve health as well as prevent
disease—also includes regular physical activity. Some health experts
recommend that adults get a minimum of 30 minutes of activity a
minimum of three to four days a week. That's only 90 minutes! Ideally,
you should get a mix of aerobic and strength exercise that averages 60
minutes a day, five days a week. You can spread the minutes out over
the day, and even over the week—if you can only get out to walk for
20 minutes at lunch, then do so five days a week to get in your minimum time.

One thing about exercise that many people don't know when they
first return to physical activity: It grows on you. Once you start walking
at lunch, you may enjoy it so much that the initial 10 minutes you
begrudgingly allotted will stretch to 20 or even 30 minutes before you
know it. It feels good to get moving. You may find your body feels
more energized and your brain is more alert. Regular exercise can make
everything seem just a little bit brighter—even you.

A word of caution: It's a good idea to get a check-up from your doctor before you begin or increase your physical activity or exercise regimen, especially if you have been inactive for a while. It's important to start with a level of activity that is right for your body. It's also important to know how you can plan activities that accommodate any health conditions you might have. Consult your doctor before beginning new sports, activities, or exercise programs.

Ask for Help if You Need It

Most of us slip into patterns of behavior without really recognizing them until we realize we're not where we want to be. If your goal is to be beef-free, but right now you have steak for dinner four nights a week, cut back one night at a time. You might find that you need two weeks before cutting back another night. You may need two months or more to completely give up steak, but that's okay. Gradual change usually makes it easier to make lasting changes. When other foods start to fill in the gap where beef once stood, you'll probably find it hard to believe you missed out on all these other wonderful foods because you were filling up on beef. The Beef Busting steps described in Chapters 13 through 16 provide you with just the guidance you need to achieve your beef-busting goal.

Of course, while this book may be a great place to start, you may need a bit more personalized attention. Talk to your doctor or dietitian for more guidance to help you make changes in eating habits, physical exercise, and general health. Beware of experts selling supplements—they often have their own, not your, best interests in mind.

If you haven't had a physical examination in the past couple of years, it's a good idea to schedule one. This will give you a clear picture of your health status and health needs. (Health experts recommend that blood cholesterol levels be checked every five years for adults.) If you don't already have a doctor, group medical practices, including health maintenance organizations (HMOs), often provide informational leaflets or brochures introducing their doctors and identifying their areas of expertise and interest. This can help you choose a doctor who shares your views about lifestyle matters and health.

Onward . . . to Change and to Better Health

The first section of this book concludes with this chapter. Our focus has been on all the whys for reducing beef in, or eliminating beef from, your diet. The following chapters focus on the hows, giving you food guidelines and recipes to make your transition to beef-free living a happy dietary adventure of health and discovery.

11

Four Steps to
Busting Beef Cravings

or any number of reasons, you have made the decision to cut back
on the beef you eat or to eliminate it entirely from your diet. But in
the end, all these reasons feed a common result: better health. From
avoiding potentially devastating illnesses spread by beef contaminated
by *Escherichia coli* or by bovine spongiform encephalopathy (BSE) to
lowering your risk for heart disease and cancer, the health benefits of
breaking away from beef are hard to ignore.

Animal-Based Foods and Illness

There is more that we *don't* know than we do know about diseases such
as mad cow disease that come to us from animal-based foods. Health
officials consider the outbreak of BSE and the resulting human form of
the disease that has occurred in Europe and some parts of Asia over the
past 15 years to be one of the worst health crises the world has known
since the end of World War II. While thousands of people have died
from influenza outbreaks, potentially millions could be infected with
the human form of mad cow disease, variant Creutzfeldt-Jakob disease
(vCJD) in a worst-case scenario.

Despite intense efforts to eradicate BSE by destroying millions of
cattle in Britain and other European countries, public health officials
worldwide continue to express concern that small pockets of contami-

nated beef supplies still exist, harboring an unknown potential to cause widespread illness. The level to which this concern affects the United States is perhaps best understood by considering the U.S. Food and Drug Administration's (FDA) recommendations. The FDA currently holds that blood donations be refused from anyone who lived in Britain for longer than 6 months between 1980 and 1996, the years during which the crisis was unfolding but was as yet undetected. People who have spent 10 years or more in France or Portugal since 1980 also are restricted from donating blood. Organizations such as the Red Cross and America's Blood Centers are calling for even tougher restrictions. The FDA is considering a proposal to extend restrictions to include donors who have lived 5 years or more in Europe since 1980, or who have spent 3 months in the United Kingdom from 1980 through the end of 1996. While there is no certainty that vCJD can be transmitted through donated blood, the FDA is concerned about the theoretical possibility and plans to re-examine safety issues and restrictions regularly for maximum protection here in the United States.

The U.S. National Institutes of Health (NIH) summarizes such concerns about the potential health risks of BSE in this statement from its report "Bovine Spongiform Encephalopathy and Variant Creutzfeldt-Jakob Disease: Background, Evolution, and Current Concerns," which appeared in the January–February 2001 issue of the journal *Emerging Infectious Diseases:*

> The epidemic of bovine spongiform encephalopathy (BSE) in the United Kingdom, which began in 1986 and has affected nearly 200,000 cattle, is waning to a conclusion, but leaves in its wake an outbreak of human Creutzfeldt-Jakob disease, most probably resulting from the consumption of beef products contaminated by central nervous system tissue. Although averaging only 10–15 cases a year since its first appearance in 1994, its future magnitude and geographic distribution (in countries that have imported infected British cattle or cattle products, or have endogenous BSE) cannot yet be predicted. The possibility that

large numbers of apparently healthy persons might be incubating the disease raises concerns about iatrogenic transmissions through instrumentation (surgery and medical diagnostic procedures) and blood and organ donations. Government agencies in many countries continue to implement new measures to minimize this risk.

While we have the perception that the beef supply in the United States, as well as throughout much of the world, is safe, the reality is that there is no way to be certain. In our modern world economy, it is foolhardy to believe that country borders or oceans can protect people and populations from the risks of disease. There is no such thing as an isolated occurrence. With a disease like BSE, symptoms can take 15 years or longer to show up; as long as new cases continue to surface, the risk continues. And at present, there is no cure for this progressive, degenerative disease—it always ends in death.

As far as researchers have been able to determine, the infectious agent (a protein substance called a prion) is confined to the brain and spinal cord tissue of an infected cow. It does not affect muscle tissue, which is the source of meat cuts such as steaks and roasts. Most health officials believe muscle tissue meats are, therefore, safe to eat in terms of being free from BSE. But modern processing methods have made it possible to use almost every shred of a slaughtered animal, increasing the likelihood for brain and especially spinal cord tissue to get into ground meat. Health officials worry that such contamination could set the stage for potential disaster.

Even in the United States, where health officials consider the beef supply to be the safest in the world, there are numerous documented circumstances of lapses in safe slaughter and handling procedures that cause great concern. U.S. Department of Agriculture (USDA) inspectors have detected spinal cord tissue in a few—very few, just 4 in 70 between 1996 and 2001—tested samples of ground meat since it began surveying for it in 1996. And none had BSE; as of 2001, no cases of BSE had been detected in the United States.

The only way to reduce your risk for experiencing the consequences of such lapses is to reduce or eliminate your exposure to them.
This means eat less, or no, beef. Will we ever have a totally safe system
for supplying beef? Probably not. There are few absolutes in life, and
there are many variables when it comes to moving food products along
the chain from source to table. A chain is only as strong—or in this
case, as healthy—as its weakest link. At present, quite a number of links
in the beef supply chain are fragile.

The Centers for Disease Control and Prevention (CDC) recommends that people traveling outside the United States, and particularly
in European and other countries where BSE has been found, take great
caution when eating beef. The CDC notes that the level of uncertainty
about BSE means that the safest approach is to avoid beef altogether. If
that is not possible or desirable, then the CDC suggests eating only beef
muscle meats certified as coming from BSE-free sources by European
health officials and avoiding ground meats, including sausages, altogether (ground meats and sausages typically contain tissues other than
muscle).

Of course, mad cow disease and the human variant Creutzfeldt-
Jakob disease are not the only public health threats that lurk within the
beef supply. Infections such as *E. coli*, salmonellosis, listeriosis, and
campylobacteriosis sicken millions of Americans every year and claim
the lives of thousands. While safe beef-handling procedures after purchase can virtually eliminate the risk from infectious pathogens that
are killed during cooking, how sure can you be about whether they've
been followed if you are not the one preparing the food? (See Chapter
2 for more on the public health risks associated with beef.)

REDUCING THE RISK FOR OTHER ILLNESS

Equally important when considering how much of a role you want
beef to play in your diet are the risks and concerns it poses for your
personal health. When beef dominates your diet, it can help set the
stage for health problems such as heart disease and cancer. Beef itself
does not cause heart disease, cancer, or other diseases, of course. It is

the amounts in which many people tend to eat beef that appear to lead to health problems.

Short and simple, most beef-eaters eat too much beef. Let's repeat this: *too much beef*. Although the recommended serving size is 3.5 ounces, the typical serving size in terms of what many Americans actually eat is anywhere from two to eight times as large. We have become accustomed to a culture of "plus size" meals, resulting in a perception that more is better. Unfortunately, however, "more" usually means more saturated fat. In fact, beef has the greatest amount of saturated fat of any of the animal meats, such as fish, poultry, veal—even pork. Too much saturated fat in the diet can increase blood cholesterol levels. And when your blood cholesterol levels climb, your risk of heart disease also increases.

When beef ceases to be the centerpiece of your meals and other plant-based foods replace the main feature of the meal, it's likely that you'll lose weight and your blood cholesterol levels will come down. Not all at once, of course, and the improvements are more marked when other health-oriented changes, such as increasing your activity level, accompany your changes in eating habits. Many health experts believe that dietary changes alone, though absolutely essential for a healthy lifestyle, are not enough. Healthy eating habits in combination with regular exercise and stress management produce the best results in terms of helping you to feel your best and supporting optimal health.

The Beef Buster Plan: Eating for Better Health

The Beef Buster plan for healthy eating includes beef-free, low-fat menus that emphasize the consumption of chronic-disease-fighting, and wonderfully satisfying plant foods. This plan provides general guidelines only. For individual dietary guidelines tailored to your specific health and personal needs, please consult with your doctor or a registered dietitian. (Many medical centers offer, or can refer you to, nutritional counseling services.)

The Beef Buster plan for healthy eating is based on the guidelines and recommendations of the USDA food pyramid and its *Dietary Guidelines for Americans*. (See Chapter 8 to view the USDA food pyramid.) We've fined-tuned those guidelines to emphasize specific foods, such as soy, that have been particularly noted to be beneficial to health from numerous scientific studies. The guidelines organize foods into categories and recommend the daily servings from each.

WHOLE GRAINS: BREAD, CEREAL, RICE, AND PASTA GROUP

The Beef Buster plan for healthy eating recommends *six or more servings a day* (depending on individual needs) from the whole-grains food group, which includes breads, cereals, rice, and pasta. One serving is equal to a single slice of whole-grain bread; a sandwich made with two slices of whole-grain bread counts as two servings. Be sure to check the calorie content for the bread you use. The standard is 70 calories per slice, so if the bread you are eating has more calories than this, you need to adjust the number of servings you eat. For example, a sandwich made with two slices of bread at 120 calories per slice is really three and one half servings, not two. By the same token, a typical bagel can count for two, and even up to six, servings! Read labels. If you are buying from a grocery store bakery or bagel store, ask for nutritional information; most have material available or can direct you to a source for providing it. This same caution applies to other foods whose calorie counts vary, such as cereals and pasta.

For other foods in this group, 70 calories count as one serving, so it's important to read the package labels. Other serving examples include ½ cup cooked whole grain (such as barley, millet, or bulgur), rice, or pasta; 1 ounce ready-to-eat cereal (amounts vary); 3 tablespoons wheat germ; ½ cup cooked cereal (such as oatmeal or farina); three or four crackers (the size of crackers varies); 1 6-inch corn tortilla; and half of an English muffin (check labels for caloric content).

Whole grains are the building blocks of sound nutrition. They contain many vitamins, minerals, and phytochemicals. Whole grain products also contain dietary fiber. When you reduce beef and increase foods such as whole grains in your diet, you will find that fiber helps you reach a feeling of fullness (satiety) during and after a meal without unwanted fat. Let's take a closer look at the grains generally available in larger grocery stores and health food markets:

- **Amaranth.** Revered by many ancient cultures including the Aztecs for its abundance and high protein. It is actually a seed and is available whole or in breads and pastas. Great as a hot cereal or side dish, either by itself or mixed with other grains.
- **Barley.** More than a sidekick for beef in soup, it is a great in other soups as well as in salads and mixed with other grains for side dishes.
- **Buckwheat.** A seed rather than a grain, it is often prepared like rice and is common in many dishes such as pancakes. Also available as groats, also known as kasha.
- **Hominy.** Commonly available as dried corn kernels with the husks removed. American southerners eat ground hominy in the form of grits. In other dishes, like stews and casseroles, it is used as a thickener. And yes, hominy comes from the same corn we also eat as a vegetable.
- **Millet.** Grown in northern Africa, this grain is rather bland in flavor, which makes it ideal for blending with other grains and foods. Good as a hot cereal or as a side dish.
- **Oats.** Whole-grain oats are a cold-morning favorite, and they are as good for you as they taste good. Buy regular oats instead of instant or quick-cooking varieties.
- **Quinoa.** From South America, quinoa is high in protein and minerals. It cooks faster than rice and is a delicious alternative as a side dish or in other dishes.
- **Rice.** There are many varieties; brown rice has more nutrients but white rice cooks faster. Good as a side dish or blended with other foods.
- **Wheat.** Perhaps the most common and versatile grain of all,

wheat is the base grain for many breads, pastas, and cereals. Look for whole-grain wheat flour, or products that contain it, for the highest nutritional value.

VEGETABLE GROUP

The Beef Busters plan for healthy eating recommends *three or more servings a day* of foods from the vegetable group. Vegetables are rich sources of vitamins, minerals, antioxidants, fiber, and phytochemicals. A serving size is one whole medium-size vegetable, 1 cup of chopped or diced raw vegetables, or ½ cup of cooked or canned vegetables.

There's no rule that says you can eat only one kind of vegetable at a time, or that vegetables can't be the main course. Many of the recipes in Chapter 16 prove the point! Try the Veggie Enchiladas with Spicy Rice or Jambalaya with Shrimp and Turkey Sausage for a new taste sensation. Include a variety of vegetables in your daily diet, to get the maximum nutrients from the many different kinds.

FRUIT GROUP

The Beef Buster meal plan recommends *at least two servings a day* from the fruit group. As with vegetables, a serving size is one whole medium-size fruit (or one small banana), 1 cup raw chopped fruit or berries, ½ cup cooked or canned (preferably canned in fruit juices only, with no added sugar), or ¼ cup dried fruit. Rich in vitamins, minerals, phytochemicals, and fiber, and naturally and wonderfully sweet, fruits make great selections when your sweet tooth screams.

LEGUMES GROUP

Often categorized with vegetables, the Beef Buster meal plan separates the legume group (beans, lentils, peas) to emphasize its unique qualities. Rich in fiber and sources of phytochemicals (like all other plant foods), they are also good sources of protein. This is a group to explore when phasing out beef from your diet and moving toward a plant-centered meal plan. Versatile and delicious, this unique treasured food group from Mother Nature offers a wide variety of textures and tastes. The Beef Buster goal for you is to eat *at least ½ cup three times per week* from the legumes group.

SOY GROUP

Technically, the soybean is a legume, but it offers so much dietary variety that we've put it in its own category to highlight its star role in disease prevention. This potent legume has been found to help to fight cancer and heart disease. The Beef Busters meal plan urges you to eat *one serving at least twice a week* from this group. Of course, the more times you can incorporate soy into your weekly eating plan, the better! Try your soy in the form of soy milk (1 cup nonfat or low-fat), soy cheese (1 ounce low-fat or nonfat), tofu (4 ounces), tempeh, and any of the textured soy products.

NUTS AND SEEDS

Nuts and seeds make up another protein food category singled out because of its wonderful benefits. Packed with fiber, phytochemicals, protein, and many vitamins and minerals, nuts and seeds are foods you will definitely want to consume on a regular basis. Even though they generally are high in fat (the chestnut is actually a low-fat food), the good fat within them is mostly in the heart-healthy monounsaturated form. The exception is the coconut, which is high in saturated fat and, therefore, should be avoided as much as possible.

The Beef Busters meal plan recommends eating a *1-ounce serving at least three times a week*. What does 1 ounce equal? About 24 almonds (165 calories), 36 peanuts (160 calories), and 4 chestnuts (80 calories). Nuts and seeds can also be enjoyed as spreads (such as 2 tablespoons of peanut butter, which equals 1 ounce), but we must emphasize the importance of eating nuts and seeds that have not been processed and that do have any added hydrogenated or partially hydrogenated oils, sodium, sugar, and/or other additives (read the labels), as is the case with many popular peanut butter brands.

Of course, you don't have to consume a 1-ounce serving at one sitting. Enjoy nuts and seeds throughout the day. For example, sprinkle

0.5 ounce on your morning cereal and enjoy another 0.5 ounce during your afternoon snack.

DAIRY GROUP

The Beef Buster meal plan recommends *at least two servings per day* of low-fat or nonfat dairy foods. Dairy foods include milk, yogurt, and cheese. Dairy foods are animal foods; therefore, the fat they contain is principally in the form of saturated fat. Choosing low-fat or nonfat varieties is best to help stave off the threat of heart disease and to save on calories, making your effort to maintain a healthy weight that much easier. Here are some examples of serving sizes: 1 cup milk, 1 cup yogurt, and 1 ounce cheese. Here's a tip: 1 ounce of cheese is about the size of your thumb, and 1 cup is about the size of your fist.

Cheeses that are considered to be higher in fat than other varieties (based on 1-ounce servings) include blue cheese, Edam, Cheddar, ricotta (made with whole milk), and brie. Lower-fat cheeses include feta, Mozzarella (made with part-skim milk), cottage cheese (made with low-fat or skim milk), Parmesan, and Romano. Luckily, just about all cheeses come in reduced-fat varieties, so even the higher-fat cheeses can be enjoyed.

Dairy foods are rich sources of calcium. Calcium is important for bone health, and getting adequate amounts throughout your life is important in reducing your risk of getting osteoporosis. Therefore, if you are eliminating dairy foods from your diet, it is important to make sure you are getting at least two servings of calcium-rich dairy alternative foods, such as calcium-fortified orange juice or calcium-fortified soy milk every day. Choose or buy only pasteurized dairy products.

ANIMAL MEATS AND EGGS GROUP

For beef-eaters, the meat group is often considered the beef group. But there are other sources of animal meats that are lower in saturated fat that can and should be enjoyed. Fish and poultry are good beef replacements. Some fish are an excellent source of omega-3 fatty acids. (See Chapter 14 for a list of fish that are high in omega-3 fatty acids.)

Always be sure to cook poultry, eggs, and fish thoroughly to reduce the risk of food-borne illness. The Beef Buster meal plan recommends the following:

- Eggs—*no more than four per week,* as recommended by the American Heart Association and the American Dietetic Association. This, of course, refers to whole eggs; egg whites, which contain no cholesterol, can be enjoyed as much as desired. Remember to count the whole eggs you use in cooking and baking.
- Fish—*one (better: two) servings per week.* Low in saturated fat, fish, especially the kinds that are high in omega-3 fatty acids, should be enjoyed weekly.
- Poultry—*one or two 3- to 4-ounce servings per week.* The Beef Busters meal planner uses poultry as a beef alternative; but it is best to get your protein from legumes, nuts and seeds, fish, and nonfat or low-fat dairy products. If you choose not to include poultry in your diet, that's okay! This is only an optional recommendation.
- Beef—*none.* This is your ultimate Beef Buster goal!

SWEETS

Sweets, like fats and oil, should make up the smallest portion of your daily diet, although for many people they compose the largest source of calories. Highly refined or processed desserts and pastries contain large amounts of saturated fat and calories and lack important disease-fighting nutrients. Candy is another food that lacks nutrients. When your sweet tooth strikes, placate it with whole fruit, fruit smoothies, frozen fruit bars, and other fruit-based treats. While an occasional sweet treat that has little nutritional value won't hurt you, it's best to keep contributions from this group to a minimum.

If you have the time, make your own desserts or sweet breads and muffins with whole grains, fruits, vegetables (such as carrot muffins or pumpkin cookies), and nuts or seeds. Be adventurous and replace the cow's milk in recipes with soy milk and the butter with olive or canola oil. Reduce the sugar and use lots of cinnamon, pure vanilla extract, and other spices. You will be surprised by the wonderful results!

ABOUT GROUND BEEF AND OTHER GROUND MEATS

The Beef Busters healthy eating plan does *not* recommend ground meats and sausages because of public health issues, such as mad cow disease and the risk for food-borne illnesses. Remember the CDC guidelines on beef consumption for European travelers given earlier in this chapter. These guidelines seem a reasonable caution for all locations given the uncertainty that surrounds BSE and its threat to human health.

Even lean ground beef—while better for you than "regular" ground beef because it's lower in fat—contains beef by-products that European health officials have outlawed. Beef and beef by-products often show up as fillers in other products, such as turkey sausage. If you choose to use ground turkey or turkey sausage as beef replacements, be sure to read the list of ingredients. If you can't tell whether the product contains any beef or beef by-products, ask the store, contact the manufacturer directly, or buy a different product you are certain is beef-free.

Planning Your Beef Busters Menu

The Beef Busters plan for healthy eating follows four steps to move you gradually and tastefully from a diet overflowing with beef to satisfying beef-free meals.

Step 1—Reduce. Examine your portion sizes and keep them to what nutritionists consider appropriate—such as 3.5-ounce cooked steak. Also, focus on reducing the higher cuts of beef in your diet, such as prime rib or regular ground beef, and replace them with the cuts that are considered to be leaner, such as loin cuts or extra-lean ground beef that you've ground at home from a solid piece of red muscle meat.

Step 2—Substitute. Begin replacing beef with other foods such as poultry and fish. Once you start to reduce beef from your diet, it's easy to find ways to replace it with other main-dish treats.

Step 3—Incorporate. Start adding some of those nutritious and delicious plant-based foods you never considered when beef dominated your diet.

Step 4—Eliminate. By now, you should be wondering why you thought beef was such a good thing in the first place.

Reducing or eliminating beef from your diet is a process of change, not a process of sacrifice. Allow yourself a reasonable amount of time to adjust to each step before moving on to the next one. After all, it's taken you a lifetime to settle into the eating habits you now have. Although it won't take another lifetime to turn to eating habits that support a healthy lifestyle, change won't happen overnight, either. But the benefits are overwhelming, from reducing your risk of food-borne illnesses to lowering your risk for the two biggest killers: heart disease and cancer. The remaining chapters take you on your four-step journey to beef-free living. Enjoy!

12

Beef Buster's
14-Day Menu Planner

A t last you've come to the culmination of the Beef Buster plan: The part where you put it all into practice. Congratulations on your progress and your continued commitment to improve your health, safety, and welfare by busting beef. If you were beginning to wonder about the safety of beef due to contamination from mad cow disease, *E. coli*, or whatever you've heard in the news before you began reading about busting beef, you are probably feeling far more committed to phasing beef out of your life now that you know so much more about it.

This menu planner will help you bring together all the ideas from this book, including the information in the first 11 chapters and the four Beef Buster steps, which are detailed in Chapters 13 through 16. But this menu planner is not meant to be a strict and rigid plan you must follow to the letter. Instead, it is meant to work with you. Based on the recipes given in the following chapters, the menu planner is a guide to help you eat well while comfortably phasing out beef and, eventually, cutting down on all meats in favor of the many varied and nutrient-dense foods available from plants.

In week 1, you'll gradually decrease the size of your beef portions, replacing the beef with other, healthier meats. In week 2, you'll add more plant foods to your diet and experiment with meatless meals. As you follow the menu planner, don't forget to drink lots of fresh, purified water; to exercise daily; and to manage your stress, keeping your entire self healthy! When a meal has no suggested beverage, please take the opportunity to have a glass of water.

For each dinner menu, you'll be given an alternate. If, while following the Beef Buster menu planner, you find you don't feel like cooking, look for one of the many prepared foods (look for packaged foods that don't contain a lot of additives) or restaurant foods that are similar to the meals suggested here. Be sure that the food you choose is as healthy as possible—fresh, low in saturated fat, and free of beef. Remember that to avoid the risk of mad cow disease, you must choose packaged foods or restaurant dishes that contain no beef, or that at least contain no ground beef, beef by-products, or sausage blends that include beef. When you do choose to eat something you don't prepare from scratch at home, be sure to read the label carefully or talk to the cook so you can feel confident that you know exactly what you are eating.

If you choose to eat ground beef, purchase muscle meat at the grocery store and grind it yourself at home on equipment you know is free of contamination. (To avoid cross-contamination of food-borne bacteria, be sure to wash your grinding equipment well after each use.) Ground turkey or chicken may be the better choice. If you're looking to turkey sausage or kielbasa as an alternative to beef sausage, be sure that the product is pure turkey and contains no beef or beef by-products (including the casings). When in doubt about the beef content of any product, read the label carefully, ask the grocer or chef, or contact the manufacturer directly. When it comes to eating ingredients you don't intend to eat or aren't comfortable eating, it's better to be safe than sorry.

One of the most wonderful and enjoyable parts of the Beef Buster program is the opportunity to learn to appreciate the magnificent variety of alternative, safer, and healthier food that is so easily available to those who are ready to find it, cook it, and savor it.

Week 1

This is the week to work on reducing your beef portion sizes and substituting other meats for beef in your menus. An asterisk after a menu item means the recipe is included in this book.

DAY 1

BREAKFAST

2 scrambled eggs

1 slice whole wheat toast

1 fresh orange

1 cup coffee, tea, or water

> NOTE: *If you are sensitive to caffeine, please discuss the safety of consuming regular coffee and other beverages containing caffeine with your doctor.*

LUNCH

Garden Steak Sandwiches*

1 apple, sliced

SNACK (OPTIONAL):

4 soda crackers

2 tablespoons peanut butter

> NOTE: *Look for peanut butter (or other "nut butters") that hasn't been processed with salt or sugar. Avoid products with hydrogenated or partially hydrogenated oil, which indicates the presence of trans fatty acids.*

1 cup milk

> NOTE: *Choose low-fat or nonfat milk. If you prefer only whole milk, that's okay at this point; but remember it's a good idea to change to low-fat or nonfat dairy products in the future.*

DINNER

Citrus-Marinated London Broil*

Smashed Potatoes*

Nutty Green Beans*

    OR

Lean Fajitas with Grilled Vegetables on Whole Wheat Tortillas*

1 cup milk

DESSERT (OPTIONAL)

1 serving warm vanilla pudding over 1 scoop of low-fat ice cream

DAY 2

BREAKFAST

1 cup oatmeal

    with walnuts, raisins, brown sugar, and milk

1 cup coffee, tea, or water

LUNCH

A Better Burger*

    NOTE: If you choose to use ground beef in this recipe, buy muscle meat and grind it yourself at home. Or, use all ground turkey.

Baked Fries*

Chopped Salad*

1 fresh pear

SNACK (OPTIONAL)

1 low-fat cereal bar

½ cup fruit juice

DINNER

Spicy Pot Roast*

Salad with Creamy Orange Dressing*

Leftover Baked Fries

OR
Tangy Beef Stroganoff*
Caesar Salad*

DESSERT (OPTIONAL)

Baked Peaches*

DAY 3

BREAKFAST

2 slices whole wheat toast
2 tablespoons all-fruit spread
1 cup milk

> NOTE: *Switch to low-fat or nonfat milk as soon as you are ready.*

1 banana

LUNCH

Meaty Pizza*

> NOTE: *Be sure that the chicken, turkey, or seafood sausage used in this pizza recipe is 100 percent pure and beef-free, including the sausage casings.*

Tossed salad with 1 tablespoon low-fat dressing
1 fresh orange

SNACK (OPTIONAL)

15 baked tortilla chips
¼ cup salsa

DINNER

Beef with Olives over Rice*
Healthy Antipasti*
OR
Shepherd's Pie*
Tossed salad with 1 tablespoon low-fat dressing

DESSERT (OPTIONAL)

Fresh Fruit Salad*

DAY 4

BREAKFAST

1 cup cold cereal with ½ cup milk
1 fresh apple
1 cup coffee, tea, or water

LUNCH

Garden Steak Sandwiches*

SNACK (OPTIONAL)

1 low-fat muffin

DINNER

Pecan-Crusted Pork Chops with Orange Sauce*
Tossed salad with 1 tablespoon low-fat dressing
Spiced Pears*
    OR
Salmon Steaks with Grilled Mushrooms and Onions*
Corn on the Cob*
Mango Slices*

DESSERT (OPTIONAL)

1 serving homemade cake with sliced fresh or canned fruit
    NOTE: Canned fruit should be packed in its own juice.

DAY 5

BREAKFAST

Fruit smoothie
    blended fresh or frozen fruit, 1 cup low-fat yogurt, and ice cubes
1 cup coffee, tea, or water

LUNCH

Turkey sandwich

whole-grain bread, turkey, low-fat cheese, lettuce, and tomato

1 apple

SNACK (OPTIONAL)

1 cup low-fat or nonfat yogurt

DINNER

Shish Kebab Barbecue*

Grilled Fruit Skewers*

OR

Chili Meat Loaf*

Homemade Coleslaw*

DESSERT (OPTIONAL)

1 cup low-fat or nonfat yogurt with fresh fruit

DAY 6

BREAKFAST

Breakfast burrito

1 scrambled egg, 1 slice low-fat cheese, and salsa rolled in a tortilla

1 cup coffee, tea, or water

LUNCH

Large green salad with 4 ounces of tuna and tomatoes

½ cup canned Mandarin oranges, packed in their own juice

SNACK (OPTIONAL)

1 slice whole wheat toast

1 tablespoon peanut butter

NOTE: Buy peanut butter that has no added ingredients.

DINNER

Roasted Tarragon Chicken*

Baked Potato*

Mixed Greens Salad*

OR

Turkey Sausage Subs*

> NOTE: *Confirm that any turkey sausage or turkey kielbasa product you bring home to your family's table is 100 percent turkey and contains no beef or beef by-products, including the sausage casings.*

DESSERT (OPTIONAL)

Banana Wheels with Milk and Honey*

DAY 7

BREAKFAST

3 small pancakes with berries and 2 tablespoons pure maple syrup

1 cup milk

LUNCH

Lentil Stew with Ham*

1 slice whole-grain bread

Tossed salad with 1 tablespoon low-fat dressing

½ cup canned peaches, packed in their own juice

SNACK (OPTIONAL)

4 cups low-fat microwave popcorn

½ cup juice

DINNER

Cheesy Rice Casserole*

Tossed salad with 1 tablespoon low-fat dressing

OR

Healthier Hash*

Tossed salad with 1 tablespoon low-fat dressing

Week 2

This week, concentrate on adding more plant foods into your meals and try going vegetarian for a few days! An asterisk after a menu item means the recipe is included in this book.

DAY 8

BREAKFAST

1 cup oatmeal
with sliced almonds, chopped dates, and ½ cup milk
NOTE: *This week, try to make the switch to low-fat or nonfat milk for you and your family.*

1 cup coffee, tea, or water

LUNCH

Fiesta Stuffed Peppers*
½ cup pinto beans
1 fresh pear

SNACK (OPTIONAL)

2 whole-grain crackers
2 tablespoons almond butter
NOTE: *Be sure that none of your nut butters contains salt, sugar, or hydrogenated oil.*

DINNER

Pepper Stir-Fry*
2 plums
    OR
Pasta Casserole with Chicken and White Beans*
Tossed salad with 1 tablespoon low-fat dressing

DESSERT (OPTIONAL)

Low-Fat Carrot-Walnut Bread*

DAY 9

BREAKFAST

1 low-fat muffin
½ grapefruit
1 cup milk

LUNCH

Red Beans and Rice*
> NOTE: *Make sure any turkey sausage product used in this recipe is beef-free, including the casings.*

Spicy Corn Muffin*
Tossed salad with 1 tablespoon low-fat dressing
1 fresh orange

SNACK (OPTIONAL)

Whole wheat pita sandwich
> *½ pita stuffed with ¼ cup chopped tomato, 1 ounce feta cheese, chopped fresh basil, and ¼ teaspoon extra-virgin olive oil*

DINNER

Salmon Stew*
1 bread stick
Tossed salad with 1 tablespoon low-fat dressing
> OR

Chef's salad
> *mixed greens, strips of chicken, shrimp, and 1 chopped hard-boiled egg*

1 bread stick

DESSERT (OPTIONAL)

Homemade Custard with Fruit*

DAY 10

BREAKFAST

1 cup cold cereal with ½ cup low-fat vanilla soy milk

½ cup cubed pineapple

1 cup coffee, tea, or water

LUNCH

Seaside Salad*

Tropical Fruit Salad*

SNACK (OPTIONAL)

1 tablespoon almonds

½ cup milk

> NOTE: *You should be used to low-fat or nonfat milk by now.*

DINNER

Chicken Pot Pie*

Tossed salad with 1 tablespoon low-fat dressing

Homemade Applesauce*

OR

Stuffed Mushrooms*

Baked Corn Fritters*

1 cup milk

DESSERT (OPTIONAL)

1 slice tropical fruit pie

DAY 11

BREAKFAST

2 low-fat waffles

2 tablespoons low-fat ricotta cheese

1 tablespoon all natural fruit syrup or pure maple syrup

1 cup milk

LUNCH

Veggie Enchiladas*

Spicy Rice*

1 cup nonfat frozen yogurt, with sliced nectarines

> *Note: If canned, choose fruit packed in its own juice, not in sugary syrup.*

SNACK (OPTIONAL)

½ cup pretzels

½ cup juice

DINNER

One-Pot Spinach Lasagna*

1 slice garlic bread

   OR

Jambalaya with Shrimp and Turkey Sausage*

> *NOTE: Confirm that any turkey sausage or turkey kielbasa product you bring home to your family's table is 100 percent turkey and contains no beef or beef by-products, including the sausage casing.*

1 slice green-chili corn bread

DESSERT (OPTIONAL)

1 apple, sliced

2 tablespoons low-fat caramel dip

DAY 12

BREAKFAST

Fruit smoothie

> *1 cup low-fat soy milk, 1 tablespoon peanut butter, 1 frozen banana*

1 cup coffee, tea, or water

Lunch

Creamy-Crunchy Egg Salad Sandwich*
Baked Carrot "Chips"*
1 kiwi, sliced

Snack (optional)

1 apple, sliced
1 ounce low-fat Cheddar cheese

Dinner

Tofu Satay with Peanut Sauce*
Raw vegetables with nonfat Ranch dip
1 cup yogurt topped with Mandarin orange sections
    OR
Artichoke Quesadillas with Capers and Cheese*
½ cup nonfat refried beans
Packaged yellow rice

Dessert (optional)

Fruit parfait

DAY 13

Breakfast

PB&J sandwich
    multigrain bread, 2 tablespoons peanut butter, 1 tablespoon all-fruit spread
1 orange
1 cup coffee, tea, or water

Lunch

Veggie wrap
    whole wheat tortilla filled with chopped fresh vegetables
1 cup nonfat yogurt

Dinner

Sesame Chicken Salad*

1 slice whole-grain bread

OR

Vegetable stew

1 to 2 cups chopped vegetables simmered in 2 cups low-fat chicken or vegetable broth

1 slice whole-grain bread

1 ounce cheese

1 fresh pear

Dessert (optional)

Fresh Fruit Salad*

DAY 14

Breakfast

Leftover Fresh Fruit Salad

1 whole-grain English muffin

2 tablespoons almond butter

1 cup coffee, tea, or water

Lunch

Veggie sandwich

whole-grain bread, sliced fresh or roasted vegetables, and nonfat cheese

2 kiwis, sliced

1 cup milk

Snack (optional)

2 rice cakes

2 tablespoons peanut butter

OR

½ cup baby carrot sticks

DINNER

Tortilla Casserole*

Tossed salad with 1 tablespoon low-fat dressing

3 tiny bananas

    OR

Holiday Stuffed Squash*

Smashed Potatoes*

½ cup cranberry sauce

DESSERT (OPTIONAL)

1 slice low-fat pumpkin pie

13

Recipes
Step 1: Reduce

t's time to take some positive action, and we've made it easy for you by helping you bust beef in four simple steps. In this chapter and each of the following three chapters, we'll explain the step, then we'll provide you with some delicious, healthful recipes to help you follow the guidelines for that step. Some recipes are grouped together to create a complete meal; other recipes are stand-alone meals all on their own. Mix. Match. Eat in good health. Look for checklists at the end of the chapters to help you monitor your progress. When you master a step, you can proceed to the next one.

The key concept for step 1 is *reduce*. The first step to busting beef in your diet is to reduce the amount of beef you eat. You can do this in two ways: by reducing the number of meals that include beef, and by reducing your portion sizes of beef at any given meal. If you find yourself eating beef almost every day, you may find it hard to believe that you can eat well with less beef, but with the recipes in this chapter, reducing your beef consumption will be easy.

Don't worry too much about busting beef completely out of your diet for now—though that's the ultimate goal. Focus on three things:

Choose lean cuts. Pick leaner rather than fattier cuts of beef. Lean beef cuts, such as the ones listed, have fewer calories, less fat, and a bit more protein per serving than high-fat beef choices like prime rib. Trim all visible fat from the beef you eat and stick with these types of beef:

- Chuck roast
- Extra-lean ground beef (But only if you grind your own! To protect fully against the potential dangers of mad cow disease, avoid processed ground beef from the grocery store, or any product that contains ground beef.)
- Eye of round roast
- Flank steak
- Round
- Sirloin
- Tenderloin

Stick to 3-ounce portion sizes. It's true that 3 ounces may not seem like a lot when you are used to a 12-ounce steak, but if you fill up on fresh vegetables, whole grains, and other healthy side dishes, you'll feel satisfied fast.

You'll also get plenty of nutrients. Americans tend to eat more protein than their bodies require. The average adult male needs 60 grams of protein each day, and the average adult female needs 50 grams. Most of us get much more than that (the average American eats around 90 grams of protein per day), so cutting down your beef portion size isn't likely to make you protein malnourished. Instead, it'll generally improve your overall health status by freeing up calories for additional nutritious plant foods and by helping you lose weight, if needed.

Don't worry about iron, either. Reducing your iron intake can cause anemia, but iron is found abundantly in plenty of other foods besides beef. Smaller beef portions also means less saturated fat, which is the kind of fat notorious for clogging arteries and contributing to poor heart health. (See Chapter 5 for more about protein and iron.)

In case you're wondering: A 3- to 4-ounce portion of beef is about the size of a deck of cards or a woman's palm; use this guide when you don't have a scale handy to weigh your meat.

Cut out one beef meal per week. If you typically eat beef seven days a week, try to cut it down to six. If you typically eat beef five days a week, try to cut it down to four. This gradual phase-out will allow you to experiment with new and different foods, broadening your culinary horizons as well as your nutritional ones. Ideally, you should also choose "organic" beef over regular beef, because it is likely to contain fewer undesirable additives, hormones, and antibiotics. Many people claim that beef from cattle raised on organic feed and not treated with hormones or antibiotics tastes fresher and more flavorful, too. The same is considered true for free-range poultry. The slightly higher price is well worth the nutritional and gastronomic benefits.

While working on step 1, remember to trim all visible fat around the edges of the cut; to cook the beef in juice or vegetable broth rather than in a lot of oil; and to keep the butter, cream, and other high-fat ingredients out of your side dishes, too. A nice lean cut of beef is great, but if you accompany it with bread buried in butter, salad drowned in creamy dressing, and a slab of cake, you'll undermine all your good efforts. And remember that to protect fully against the dangers of mad cow disease avoid products that contain beef sausage. Ground beef is off limits as well, unless you buy a steak or other piece of muscle meat, trim the fat, and grind the meat yourself in a professional grade food processor.

If you need some additional inspiration, take a look at the following recipes for filling meals that contain no more than 3 ounces of lean beef per serving. (It's really enough food!) Pick the ones that sound good or try them all. You'll discover that you can learn to live without as much beef as you're used to, and before long, you'll be able to get beef out of your diet altogether. While eating lean cuts, reducing your portion size of beef, and also reducing the number of beef servings per week are great ways to eat more healthfully, avoiding products that contain any beef or beef by-products is the safest way to protect against the potential dangers of mad cow disease. (See Chapter 2 for more about mad cow disease.)

RECIPES

Citrus-Marinated London Broil
with Smashed Potatoes and Nutty Green Beans

This meal is high on flavor but low on fat. Skip the fatty sauce tradition-ally served with London broil: Slice your meat thinly across the grain and serve it with orange wedges to squeeze over the top. The flavor intensity from the citrus is so satisfying that you don't need much; you'll find that 3 ounces of beef is plenty, especially when the rest of your plate is loaded with creamy (but low-fat) potatoes and nutty-good green beans.

CITRUS-MARINATED LONDON BROIL

SERVES 4

> *12 ounces extra-lean top round or eye round roast*
> *Salt and freshly ground black pepper, to taste*
> *3 tablespoons freshly squeezed orange juice*
> *3 tablespoons freshly squeezed grapefruit juice*
> *3 tablespoons freshly squeezed lemon juice*
> *1 tablespoon red wine or cider vinegar*
> *1 teaspoon extra-virgin olive oil*
> *1 tablespoon finely chopped onion*
> *1 garlic clove chopped or put through a press*
> *½ teaspoon crushed dried oregano*
> *¼ teaspoon sweet paprika*
> *1 garlic clove, thinly sliced*
> *Orange wedges, for serving*

Score both sides of the roast with a sharp knife in a criss-cross pat-tern, cutting about ¼ inch deep. Rub both sides with salt and pepper. Put the meat into a large, sealable plastic bag. Wash your hands.

In a small bowl, combine all remaining ingredients, except the sliced garlic and orange wedges, and mix. Pour the marinade into the bag over meat, seal, and refrigerate. Let the beef marinate for 2 to 6 hours.

Preheat the broiler. Spray a broiler pan with nonstick cooking spray.

Remove the roast from the bag and discard the remaining marinade. Pat the roast dry with paper towels. Randomly place slices of garlic inside the cuts on the top side of the meat. Broil about 4 inches below the heat, about 15 minutes for every inch the meat is thick, or until done (use a meat thermometer to check that the roast is fully cooked). Flip the meat over after the first 10 minutes of broiling.

To serve, slice the roast thinly with a sharp, serrated knife and serve 3-ounce portions with juicy wedges of orange.

Nutritional information per serving: 108 calories, 4 grams total fat (1 gram saturated, 2 grams monounsaturated), 18 grams protein, 0 grams fiber, 2 milligrams iron, 38 milligrams cholesterol, 42 milligrams sodium

SMASHED POTATOES

SERVES 4

> *4 medium red potatoes, eyes removed with a sharp knife*
> *¼ cup nonfat buttermilk*
> *¼ cup nonfat plain yogurt*
> *2 ounces nonfat cream cheese*
> *2 ounces low-fat Cheddar cheese, shredded*
> *Low-fat or nonfat milk or additional buttermilk, to achieve desired consistency*
> *Salt and freshly ground black pepper, to taste*
> *Sweet paprika, to taste*

Boil the potatoes whole in a large saucepan in enough water to cover them well (although they will float), until fork-tender, 20 to 30 minutes, depending on size.

Drain the potatoes and put into a large bowl. Using a knife and fork, cut each potato into four to six pieces to break up the skins. With a potato masher, smash the potatoes until chunky. Add the buttermilk, yogurt, and cheeses and continue mashing until the mixture is uniform. If the potatoes seem too stiff or dry, add enough low-fat milk to make the mixture creamy. Season with salt, pepper, and paprika.

Nutritional information per serving: 148 calories, 1 gram total fat (0.6 gram saturated, 0 gram monounsaturated), 11 grams protein, 3 grams fiber, 1 milligram iron, 4 milligrams cholesterol, 293 milligrams sodium

NUTTY GREEN BEANS

SERVES 4

> *1 pound fresh green beans, ends snapped off and strings removed,*
>   *if desired*
> *1 teaspoon extra-virgin olive oil*
> *¼ cup total sliced almonds and chopped walnuts*
> *¼ teaspoon hot red pepper flakes*

Boil the green beans in a large saucepan in enough salted water to cover until almost fork-tender, about 15 minutes.

Drain the beans and add to a large, heated skillet brushed with the olive oil. Sauté for about 5 minutes over medium-high heat, then add the nuts and red pepper flakes. Sauté another 3 minutes. Serve hot.

Nutritional information per serving: 110 calories, 7 grams total fat (0.7 gram saturated, 2 grams monounsaturated), 4 grams protein, 4 grams fiber, 0 milligram cholesterol, 2 milligrams iron, 4 milligrams sodium

LEAN FAJITAS WITH GRILLED VEGETABLES
ON WHOLE WHEAT TORTILLAS

Steak fajitas are a favorite among lovers of Mexican cuisine, but with loads of steak, cheese, and sour cream, the fat, cholesterol, and calories really add up. In this satisfying version, just a few flavorful strips of lean beef cooked without oil give the fajitas a meaty taste, but the vegetables are the real stars, contributing to the grilled flavor and making this a filling and nutrient-dense main course.

SERVES 4

12 ounces (¼-inch-thick) lean steak, such as beef roast-eye round,
    fat trimmed
1 cup beef broth (to avoid processed beef products substitute
    chicken or vegetable broth, or water)
¼ cup Worcestershire sauce
1 medium yellow onion, thickly sliced
1 medium green bell pepper, cut into ½-inch-wide strips
1 medium red bell pepper, cut into ½-inch-wide strips
2 large Portobello mushroom caps, thickly sliced
8 (12-inch) whole wheat tortillas
4 cups fresh torn lettuce leaves
1 large or 2 medium ripe tomatoes, sliced
Salsa, purchased or homemade, to taste
Nonfat sour cream, to taste

Pound the steak on both sides with a mallet to tenderize it; then slice it thinly across the grain into 24 strips (6 for each person).

In a large skillet, heat the broth and Worcestershire sauce over medium heat. When hot, add the beef strips. Simmer, turning occasionally, until the beef is cooked through, 15 to 20 minutes.

Meanwhile, spray the cooking grate of an outside grill or a stovetop grill with nonstick cooking spray. Preheat the grill. Also preheat the oven to 200°F.

Grill the onions, bell peppers, and mushrooms until tender, brushing with extra Worcestershire sauce, if desired.

Wrap the tortillas in foil and heat in the oven for about 10 minutes, or until hot.

To serve, top each tortilla with 3 strips of beef, allowing two tortillas per person. Arrange the grilled vegetables on a platter and place the lettuce, tomatoes, salsa, and sour cream in dishes for individual fajita assembly.

Nutritional information per serving: 366 calories, 6 grams total fat (2 grams saturated, 3 grams monounsaturated), 30 grams protein, 8 grams fiber, 47 milligrams cholesterol, 5 milligrams iron, 1069 milligrams sodium

NOTE: To reduce the sodium in this recipe, use low-sodium broth and reduce the amount of Worcestershire sauce, adding freshly ground black pepper for flavoring.

Spicy Pot Roast, Salad with Creamy Orange Dressing, and Baked Sweet Potato Fries

The spicy flavoring of this pot roast helps a little meat go a long way. Cool the heat with crisp mixed greens drizzled with creamy (but low-fat) orange-flavored dressing. The satisfying sweetness of sweet potatoes makes dessert unnecessary.

SPICY POT ROAST

SERVES 4

> *2 tablespoons unbleached all-purpose flour*
> *12-ounce boneless lean beef roast, such as eye of round roast, cut into four pieces*
> *1 teaspoon extra-virgin olive oil*
> *1 cup beef broth (or substitute chicken or vegetable broth, or water), plus an extra ¼ cup if needed*
> *1 (16-ounce) jar purchased salsa or 2 cups homemade*
> *1 green bell pepper, cut into large chunks*
> *1 medium yellow onion, cut into large chunks*

Put the flour in a small bowl and dredge the pieces of roast in it until they are completely covered.

Spray a large saucepan or a Dutch oven lightly with nonstick cooking spray; then add the olive oil. Heat over medium heat just until you notice the oil's aroma, about 3 minutes. Brown the meat on all sides. Add ½ cup of the broth and the salsa and bring to a simmer; then lower the heat to medium-low and cover the pan with a tight-fitting lid. Cook 30 minutes.

Add the green pepper and onion, stirring to coat with the salsa mixture. If the pot roast looks dry, add the remaining beef broth. Cover and cook another 30 minutes, or until meat is done (no pink, use a meat thermometer to ensure the meat is fully cooked).

Remove the meat and vegetables from the pan. Add just enough broth or water to the remaining salsa mixture to make a thick sauce (you may not need to add any liquid). Stir and heat through. Serve the sauce on the side.

Nutritional information per serving: 258 calories, 14 grams total fat (5 grams saturated, 2 grams monounsaturated), 20 grams protein, 2 grams fiber, 52 milligrams cholesterol, 2 milligrams iron, 951 milligrams sodium

NOTE: Use low-sodium broth to reduce sodium content in this recipe.

SALAD WITH CREAMY ORANGE DRESSING

SERVES 8

1 cup low-fat vanilla yogurt
½ cup freshly squeezed orange juice
1 garlic clove finely chopped or put through a press
1 teaspoon fresh dill or ½ teaspoon dried
¼ teaspoon salt
8 cups mixed greens

Put the yogurt, orange juice, garlic, dill, and salt into a jar with a tight-fitting lid. Cover and shake until thoroughly combined. Serve over the mixed greens. Store extra in the refrigerator up to 3 days.

Nutritional information per serving: 47 calories, 0.5 gram total fat (0.2 gram saturated, 0.9 gram monounsaturated), 2 grams protein, 1 gram fiber, 2 milligrams cholesterol, 1 milligram iron, 67 milligrams sodium

BAKED SWEET POTATO FRIES

SERVES 4

> *2 large or 4 medium sweet potatoes*
> *Salt to taste*

Preheat the oven to 400°F. Spray a large baking sheet with nonstick cooking spray.

Peel the sweet potatoes and cut them into strips, about ½ inch thick. Arrange the strips in the prepared pan so they aren't touching and spray lightly with nonstick cooking spray. Bake about 30 minutes, or until the potatoes are tender and lightly browned. Salt to taste.

Nutritional information per serving: 117 calories, 0 gram total fat, 2 grams protein, 3 grams fiber, 0 milligram cholesterol, 0.5 milligram iron, 0 milligram sodium (if no salt is used for flavor)

Tangy Beef Stroganoff with Caesar Salad and Baked Peaches

Beef stroganoff is comfort food, but its traditional richness isn't in line with smart eating practices. Try this version instead: All the warmth, comfort, and creaminess you remember, but hardly any of the fat. Stroganoff is traditionally served over hot cooked egg noodles, but it makes a fine sauce for any type of pasta, and it's pretty good over toast, too. Or, enjoy it all by itself . . . with a spoon! A crisp Caesar salad made with low-fat or nonfat dressing and tuna in place of the notorious anchovies and warm baked peaches round out a meal that will make you feel supremely satisfied.

TANGY BEEF STROGANOFF

SERVES 4

> *¼ cup reduced-sodium soy sauce*
> *¼ cup Port, dry sherry, dark beer, or red wine vinegar*
> *12 ounces sirloin, trimmed of all visible fat and cut against the*
> *grain into thin strips*
> *4 ounces nonfat sour cream*
> *2 tablespoons all-purpose flour*

¼ cup beef broth (or substitute chicken or vegetable broth,
    or water)
½ teaspoon ground cumin
½ teaspoon crushed dried oregano
8 ounces fresh mushrooms, sliced
1 medium onion, chopped
2 garlic cloves, minced or put through a press
4 ounces nonfat yogurt
Chopped fresh parsley or cilantro, for garnish

Mix the soy sauce and Port in a medium bowl. Add the beef strips and marinate, covered with plastic wrap, in the refrigerator for 30 to 60 minutes. In another bowl, mix the sour cream, flour, broth, cumin, and oregano; set aside.

Spray a large nonstick skillet with nonstick cooking spray and place over medium-high heat. Pour the meat and marinade into the skillet and cook until meat is done (no pink, use a meat thermometer to ensure that the meat is fully cooked), about 3 minutes. Remove the meat with a slotted spoon and set aside.

Add the mushrooms, onion, and garlic to the skillet. Sauté until the vegetables begin to soften. Return the meat to the skillet and add the sour cream mixture. Reduce heat to medium and cook, stirring constantly, until the mixture is thick and bubbly. Reduce heat to medium-low and stir in the yogurt. Sprinkle with parsley and serve.

Nutritional information per serving: 210 calories, 4 grams total fat (1 gram saturated, 1 gram monounsaturated), 16 grams protein, 2 grams fiber, 54 milligrams cholesterol, 33 milligrams iron, 1219 milligrams sodium

NOTE: Reduce the sodium content in this recipe by using low-sodium broth, or by reducing the amount of soy sauce used.

CAESAR SALAD

SERVES 4

8 cups bite-size pieces of torn Romaine lettuce leaves
½ cup nonfat plain yogurt
½ cup nonfat sour cream
¼ cup beef broth (or substitute chicken or vegetable broth,
    or water)
1 tablespoon tuna packed in olive oil
1 tablespoon freshly squeezed lemon juice
1 tablespoon grated Parmesan cheese
1 garlic clove
¼ teaspoon freshly ground black pepper
1 slice good whole wheat or multigrain bread
½ teaspoon extra-virgin olive oil

Preheat the oven to 400°F.

Put the lettuce in a large salad bowl.

Put the yogurt, sour cream, broth, tuna, lemon juice, cheese, garlic, and pepper in a blender jar; cover and blend until smooth.

Brush the bread with the olive oil and toast in the oven on a baking sheet for about 5 minutes on each side, or until brown and crisp. Cut the toast into 16 cubes.

Toss ½ cup of the dressing and toast cubes with the lettuce until coated. Store the remaining dressing in the refrigerator for up to 3 days.

Nutritional information per serving: 92 calories, 3 grams total fat (0.5 gram saturated fat, 0.3 gram monounsaturated fat), 7 grams protein, 1 gram fiber, 4 milligrams cholesterol, 2 milligrams iron, 269 milligrams sodium (or about 220 milligrams sodium if water is used instead of broth)

BAKED PEACHES

Serves 4

4 firm ripe peaches
1 cup dry breadcrumbs or graham cracker crumbs
½ cup packed light brown sugar
1 teaspoon ground cinnamon
½ teaspoon ground nutmeg
1 tablespoon freshly squeezed lemon juice
1 tablespoon plus ½ cup freshly squeezed orange juice
2 teaspoons extra-virgin olive oil
1 tablespoon honey
2 cups low-fat vanilla yogurt, refrigerated or frozen (optional)

Preheat the oven to 350°F.

Cut the peaches in half and remove the pits. Place the halves cut side up in a casserole or a baking dish large enough to hold them without touching.

In a small bowl, mix the breadcrumbs, sugar, cinnamon, and nutmeg. Spoon one-eighth of the crumb mixture into the center of each peach half.

Mix the lemon juice with 1 tablespoon of the orange juice, and drizzle a little over the top of each peach half. Drizzle the peaches with the olive oil and then with the honey.

Mix the remaining ½ cup orange juice with ½ cup water. Pour carefully into the bottom of the dish, using just enough to come about a third of the way up the side of the peaches. Put the pan carefully into the oven and cover with the lid or aluminum foil. Bake 20 minutes. Remove the cover and bake another 5 to 10 minutes, or until the peaches are soft and topping is lightly browned.

Serve with yogurt, if desired.

Nutritional information per serving: 437 calories, 6 grams total fat (2 grams saturated fat, 1 gram monounsaturated fat), 11 grams protein, 4 grams fiber, 6 milligrams cholesterol, 3 milligrams iron, 325 milligrams sodium

Beef with Olives over Rice and Healthy Antipasti

This meal is a little light on the beef but is very filling and high in flavor. You can use any olives for this recipe, but Greek olives (such as kalamata olives) are typically better than the ubiquitous "Spanish" olives that aren't really from Spain. Whatever olives you use, they create a flavor bridge to the antipasti, which is a marinated salad.

BEEF WITH OLIVES OVER RICE

SERVES 4

> *12 ounces beef tenderloin, fat trimmed and cut into bite-size pieces*
> *12 olives pitted and cut in half*
> *¼ cup balsamic vinegar*
> *½ cup beef broth (or substitute chicken or vegetable broth, or water)*
> *1 tablespoon soy sauce*
> *2 tablespoons all-purpose flour*
> *1 teaspoon crushed dried basil*
> *¼ teaspoon hot red pepper flakes, or to taste (optional)*
> *2 cups hot cooked brown long-grain or basmati rice*

Heat a large nonstick skillet over medium heat. Add all ingredients except rice and combine thoroughly. Cook, stirring occasionally, until the sauce is slightly thickened and bubbly, and the meat is cooked through, about 30 minutes.

Spoon each serving over ½ cup of the rice.

Nutritional information per serving (including the rice): 390 calories, 21 grams total fat (8 grams saturated, 0 gram monounsaturated), 20 grams protein, 3 grams fiber, 3 milligrams iron, 60 milligrams cholesterol, 659 milligrams sodium

NOTE: To reduce the sodium in this recipe, use low-sodium broth and reduced-sodium soy sauce.

HEALTHY ANTIPASTI

Serves 4

8 ounces mushrooms, sliced

1 (4-ounce) jar marinated artichoke hearts

1 red bell pepper or 1 (4-ounce) jar roasted red bell peppers, cut into 1-inch strips

½ green or other color bell pepper, cut into 1-inch strips

8 cherry or grape tomatoes, halved or quartered

4 olives, pitted and quartered

1 garlic clove, minced or put through a press

4 ounces part-skim Mozzarella cheese, cut into small dice

1 tablespoon extra-virgin olive oil

¼ cup tarragon, white wine, or cider vinegar

¼ teaspoon crushed dried oregano

¼ teaspoon crushed dried basil

Mix all ingredients in a large bowl. Cover and allow to marinate in the refrigerator for 1 to 24 hours. The longer the salad marinates, the more the flavors mingle and intensify.

Nutritional information: 185 calories, 11 grams total fat (4 grams saturated, 5 grams monounsaturated), 2 grams fiber, 15 milligrams cholesterol, 1 milligram iron, 321 milligrams sodium

GARDEN STEAK SANDWICHES

These sandwiches are excellent picnic fare as long as the mayonnaise is kept chilled. Make this recipe when produce is at its freshest from your garden, the farmers market, or the local grocer. Feel free to add more vegetables to your sandwich (adding more dietary fiber—a good thing!), but keep the beef to 2 ounces.

Serves 4

4 tablespoons nonfat mayonnaise

1 teaspoon spicy brown mustard

½ teaspoon chili powder

8 thick slices fresh dark rye bread or 8 whole wheat sub rolls
¼ cup shredded carrots
8 thin slices Vidalia or other sweet onion
8 thick slices beefsteak or other large, hearty red tomato
8 large dark green lettuce leaves, dried
8 thin green, red, orange, or yellow bell pepper rings
8 thin cucumber slices
8 dill pickle slices
1 cup raw or lightly sautéed sliced mushrooms
8 ounces thinly sliced lean roast beef from the deli

In a small bowl, combine the mayonnaise, mustard, and chili powder. Spread one-eighth of the mixture evenly on each bread slice.

Line up four slices of the bread. Divide the shredded carrots evenly on top of each slice (the mayonnaise will help keep them in place), then add the other vegetables in whatever amount you like. Top each sandwich with 2 ounces of roast beef and the final piece of bread.

To serve, press each sandwich gently to secure and cut in half. Serve with lemonade and baked tortilla chips.

Nutritional information per sandwich: 376 calories, 8 grams total fat (3 grams saturated, 3 grams monounsaturated), 24 grams protein, 9 grams fiber, 45 milligrams cholesterol, 5 grams iron, 770 milligrams sodium

Shepherd's Pie with Fresh Fruit Salad

Technically, shepherd's pie is made with ground lamb; the dish made with ground beef is really called cottage pie. Because we're already taking liberties with the name, let's substitute some ground turkey to give this dish an even more interesting flavor. You can have your ground beef in this recipe only if you grind your own. Buy a lean cut of red muscle meat, trim the fat, and grind the meat in a professional grade food processor. Packaged ground beef from the supermarket is off limits if you want to get protection against the dangers of mad cow disease. To achieve the best protection—it's totally turkey time; use ground turkey in this recipe in place of lean ground beef. Be sure that the turkey is ground on machinery that only grinds turkey—and not beef as well! Fresh fruit is a nice, light finish for this warm, hearty stew-like dish.

SHEPHERD'S PIE

SERVES 4

> *2 pounds potatoes, peeled, rinsed, and quartered*
> *½ cup low-fat buttermilk*
> *4 ounces nonfat cream cheese*
> *½ teaspoon salt*
> *6 ounces extra-lean ground beef (only if you grind your own!)*
> *6 ounces lean ground turkey breast (or make the whole 12 ounces*
>   *ground turkey and eliminate the ground beef from this recipe)*
> *2 bay leaves*
> *½ teaspoon ground nutmeg*
> *¼ teaspoon ground cloves*
> *1 teaspoon dried thyme*
> *1 teaspoon freshly ground black pepper*
> *1 cup sliced carrots*
> *1 cup sliced onion*
> *1 cup sliced celery*
> *1 cup sliced mushrooms*
> *1 tablespoon all-purpose flour*
> *1 cup beef broth (or substitute chicken or vegetable broth, or water)*
> *1 tablespoon shredded part-skim Mozzarella cheese*

Boil the potatoes for about 15 minutes or until tender. Drain. Place the potatoes in a medium bowl and add the buttermilk, cream cheese, and salt. Mash with a potato masher or use a hand-held mixer set to "low" or "stir." Set aside.

Preheat the oven to 400°F.

Spray a large nonstick skillet with nonstick cooking spray. Add the ground beef (if using) and ground turkey and brown over medium heat, breaking the meat up with a spoon or spatula as it cooks. This takes about 10 to 15 minutes. Drain off the fat. Add the bay leaves, nutmeg, cloves, thyme, black pepper, carrots, onions, celery, and mushrooms. Cook, stirring, for about 2 minutes over medium heat. Add the flour and stir to coat. Mix in the broth. Cook until bubbly; then reduce the heat to a simmer and stir until thickened, about 10 minutes.

Pour the meat mixture into a 9-inch pie plate or 8-inch-square baking pan. Spoon the mashed potatoes on top, covering the meat mixture completely and sealing the pie at the edges of the pan. Sprinkle the potatoes with the cheese. Bake 30 minutes, or until casserole is heated through, potatoes are golden, and cheese is melted. Cool 10 minutes. Cut the pie into four pieces and serve.

Nutritional information per serving: 418 calories, 9 grams total fat (3 grams saturated, 3 monounsaturated), 30 grams protein, 6 grams fiber, 55 milligrams cholesterol, 5 milligrams iron, 922 milligrams sodium

NOTE: To reduce the sodium in this recipe, use low-sodium broth.

FRESH FRUIT SALAD

SERVES 4

> *2 cups bite-size pieces of fresh fruit*
> *1 tablespoon freshly squeezed lemon juice*
> *1 tablespoon freshly squeezed orange juice*
> *1 tablespoon sugar*

Put the fruit in a bowl and drizzle with the juices. Sprinkle in the sugar and stir to coat. Let sit at room temperature for 15 to 30 minutes to allow the sugar to work its magic of drawing out the fruit's natural flavor. Serve in bowls drizzled with a little of the juice.

Nutritional information per serving: 57 calories, 0 gram total fat, 2 grams fiber, 0.6 grams protein, 0 milligram cholesterol, 2 milligrams sodium

NOTE: Use whatever fruit and in whatever combination you'd like, including strawberries, blueberries, blackberries, raspberries, apples, pears, peaches, nectarines, plums, apricots, oranges, tangerines, bananas, cantaloupe, honeydew, watermelon, kiwi, mango, papaya, and pineapple.

MONITOR YOUR PROGRESS—STEP 1

❏   I am choosing only the leanest cuts of beef.

❏   I am limiting my beef portions to 3 ounces.

❏   I am reducing the number of days each week I include beef in my meal plans.

❏   I am buying beef from cattle raised on organic feed and not treated with hormones, antibiotics, or other additives.

❏   I am only eating extra-lean ground beef that I've ground myself at home using a professional grade food processor—no store-bought ground beef.

❏   I am substituting chicken or vegetable broth (or just plain water) for beef broth when called for in recipes.

Once you've mastered step 1, proceed to step 2.

14

Recipes
Step 2: Substitute

Now that you've mastered portion size reduction and are choosing leaner cuts of beef, you can move on to step 2: *substitution*. In this chapter, we'll help you begin substituting other kinds of meats—fish, chicken, turkey, and lean pork—for the beef you were once eating.

Alternative lean meats are often smarter nutritional choices than beef. Other kinds of meat, especially certain kinds of fish, contain higher amounts of omega-3 fatty acids than beef. These other meats also tend to contain lower amounts of saturated fat than beef and often contain fewer calories as well.

Generally, from a nutritional point of view, meats are divided into four categories: extra-lean, lean, medium fat, and high fat. In the last chapter, we worked on including cuts of beef from the lean categories rather than the higher-fat categories. In this chapter, we'll focus more on choosing meats other than beef from the lean and very lean categories, such as white-meat chicken and turkey without the skin, salmon, tuna, shrimp, and lean cuts of pork. These meats also tend to have lower amounts of saturated fat than beef.

When it comes to calories, choosing leaner and non-beef cuts of meat is also beneficial. In general, very lean meats will help you save on calories. For example, skinless white-meat chicken and turkey contain about 35 calories per ounce, whereas a lean cut of steak contains about 55 calories per ounce. Now, 20 calories may not seem like a lot, but when you multiply that times your 4-ounce portion, you've suddenly got 80 calories. Multiply that times 10 meals a week, and you'll save 800 calories in a week, just by substituting! If you are used to eating higher-fat cuts of meat, such as prime rib that's even been trimmed of all visible fat around the edges, you'll save 1,600 calories per week by switching to skinless white-meat chicken or turkey! What a difference. And you can double that savings again if you typically consume high-fat meats. It takes 3,500 calories to make 1 pound of body fat, so if you were to switch from high-fat meat to very lean meat twice a day, you could technically lose about 1 pound of fat a week without doing anything else differently.

Of course, weight loss is really determined by how many calories you use in relation to how many calories you eat. To better understand your individual caloric needs and to achieve and maintain a healthy weight for you, please seek the advice of a registered dietitian or other qualified health-care professional.

Omega-3 fatty acids are another important consideration when figuring out which meats you should use when substituting for beef. These are the fats you really want to get into your diet. Many studies demonstrate the profound benefits of omega-3 fatty acids on heart health, vascular health, and even brain health. The best meat sources of omega-3s are fish, and the fish with the highest amounts of omega-3s are listed in the table, along with other foods that naturally contain these beneficial fatty acids.

While working through this chapter, keep in mind that substitution can make a big difference in your health. When you get a craving for beef, consider what you might eat instead. The recipes in this chapter give you some great options. Some recipes fit together as meals; others are meals in themselves.

OMEGA-3 FATTY ACIDS

Food Item	Omega-3 Fatty Acids (grams)
Mackerel, Atlantic (3.5 ounces)	2.60
Trout, lake (3.5 ounces)	2.00
Walnuts, English/Persian (1 ounce)	1.90
Herring, Atlantic (3.5 ounces)	1.70
Tuna, albacore (3.5 ounces)	1.50
Salmon, Atlantic (3.5 ounces)	1.40
Bluefish (3.5 ounces)	1.20
Cod liver oil (1 teaspoon)	0.90
Soybeans, green (1 ounce raw)	0.90
Trout, rainbow (3.5 ounces)	0.60
Beans, common (3.5 ounces dry)	0.60
Canola oil (1 teaspoon)	0.52
Soybeans (1 ounce dry)	0.50
Kale (3.5 ounces raw)	0.20
Wheat germ (1 tablespoon)	0.10
Avocado, California (3.5 ounces)	0.10
Strawberries (3.5 ounces raw)	0.10
Broccoli (3.5 ounces raw)	0.10

SOURCE: Adapted from Mahan, Kathleen and Sylvia Escott-Stump. *Krause's Food, Nutrition, & Diet Therapy,* 9th ed. (Philadelphia: Saunders, 1996).

RECIPES

Salmon Steaks with Grilled Mushrooms and Onions, Corn on the Cob, and Mango Slices

Beef lovers may despair at the thought of giving up the whole summer barbecue tradition. What's a barbecue without a couple of T-bones, or at least some thick, juicy burgers? But the grill is actually a highly versatile piece of equipment, and many meats (and vegetables, too) taste fantastic when cooked on the grill. One of the best alternatives is salmon, which is not only lower in calories than that T-bone but supplies your body with a rich dose of heart-healthy omega-3 fatty acids, something you won't find in today's domesticated beef. Smothered in grilled mushrooms and onions, salmon steaks are just as satisfying as beef steaks. Add corn on the cob for the sake of a delicious tradition, but forget the butter. Flavor it with chili powder and fresh limes instead. Sliced mango makes for an exotic and fla-vorful finish to a nutrient-dense and extra-delicious dinner straight from the grill.

SALMON STEAKS WITH GRILLED MUSHROOMS AND ONIONS

SERVES 4

> 1 tablespoon extra-virgin olive oil
> 2 tablespoons freshly squeezed lemon or orange juice
> 4 (1-inch-thick) salmon steaks or filets
> 2 medium yellow onions, thickly sliced
> 8 ounces mushrooms, cut in half
> 2 lemons or oranges, quartered

Spray the grill grate with cooking spray and preheat the grill according to the manufacturer's instructions.

Mix the olive oil and lemon juice in a small bowl. Brush the salmon, onions, and mushrooms lightly on both sides with oil mixture and place on the grill. Cook, uncovered, about 5 minutes. Turn the fish and vegetables, brushing all with more oil mixture. Cook until the salmon flakes easily and vegetables are tender, about 5 minutes more.

Serve the salmon topped with the vegetables. Garnish each with two lemon wedges.

Nutritional information per serving: 444 calories, 15 grams total fat (2 grams saturated, 2 grams monounsaturated), 65 grams protein, 2 grams fiber, 3 milligrams iron, 165 milligrams cholesterol, 217 milligrams sodium

CORN ON THE COB

You can boil the corn or even grill it (remove the silk if grilling), but microwaving is actually a quick, easy, and highly flavorful way to cook corn on the cob. The microwave steams the corn right in the husk, bringing out its sweetness.

SERVES 4

4 medium ears of corn in the husks
4 sprigs cilantro
2 limes, quartered
Chili powder, for serving

Peel down one husk leaf on each ear of corn and insert a sprig of cilantro below the silk. Replace the husk. If the husk is loose, tie it with kitchen twine. Place the corn on the bottom of the microwave like spokes of a wheel, small ends in the center. Microwave on high for 10 minutes.

Let the corn sit for about 5 minutes; then, using oven mitts and extreme caution (the corn will still be very hot), remove the corn from the microwave and peel off the husks. Serve with lime wedges for rubbing over the corn and chili powder for sprinkling over the lime juice.

Nutritional information per serving: 70 calories, 0.5 gram total fat (0.1 gram saturated, 0.2 gram monounsaturated), 2 grams protein, 3 grams fiber, 0.5 milligram iron, 0 milligram cholesterol, 6 milligrams sodium

MANGO SLICES

Most of the people who don't like mango haven't actually tried it, or they have eaten only bad ones. Mangoes are at their best in June (the perfect time for a barbecue). Pick firm, fat fruits without blemishes or bruises and without a gray tinge. Under-ripe mangoes will ripen uncovered in a cool room or in a paper bag. Ripe mangoes have a heady aroma and feel tender to the touch.

SERVES 4

> *4 ripe mangoes*
> *1 orange, preferably organic*

Slice through the mangoes the long way twice, quartering them. Peel off the skin and cut the fruit away from the pit with a sharp knife. Put the mango slices in a large bowl. Grate the zest from the orange and sprinkle over the mangoes; then squeeze the juice over the fruit. Chill for 30 minutes to 2 hours. Serve in chilled, frosted glass dessert dishes or salad bowls for a special touch.

Nutritional information per serving: 156 calories, 0.6 gram total fat (0.1 gram saturated, 0.2 gram monounsaturated), 1.5 grams protein, 5 grams fiber, 0 milligram iron, 0 milligram cholesterol, 4 milligrams sodium

MEATY PIZZA WITH ONIONS, GARLIC, MUSHROOMS, PEPPERS, AND OLIVES

This hearty pizza, served with a green salad, makes a satisfying meal that doesn't take too long to make because it uses a purchased pizza crust. If you have extra time, you can make your own crust, but this method is a lot faster. This dish gives you all of the flavor and texture of a meat pizza without any of the beef. Feel free to substitute or change the amounts of the vegetables and the mix of meats. For example, ground or chunked chicken breast can stand in for the turkey. The Salad with Creamy Orange Dressing (recipe included in Chapter 13) goes well with this pizza.

SERVES 4

> *1 purchased pizza crust (such as Boboli), about 12 inches in diameter*
> *½ pound ground turkey breast*

2 ounces chicken, turkey, or seafood sausage (all sausage products,
*   including the casings, must be 100 percent beef-free—no beef*
*   blends)*
1 cup sliced fresh mushrooms
1 medium yellow onion, chopped
4 garlic cloves, minced
½ cup tomato sauce
½ teaspoon crushed dried oregano
2 ounces turkey ham, cut into small squares or triangles
½ teaspoon crushed dried basil
1 cup chopped green or red bell pepper
1 (4-ounce) can sliced black olives, drained and rinsed
8 ounces part skim Mozzarella cheese, shredded
¼ teaspoon dried crushed tarragon

Preheat oven to 400°F. Spray the pizza crust lightly with cooking spray and put it on a pizza pan, cookie sheet, or pizza stone.

Put the turkey breast and sausage in a bowl and, using your hands, combine well. Heat a large nonstick skillet over medium heat. Add the meat mixture. Cook until brown, breaking it apart with a spatula or wooden spoon. Drain off the fat and set the pan aside. Put the meat on a double layer of paper towels and cover it with more paper towels to soak up any additional fat.

Add the mushrooms, onions, and garlic to the pan and sauté over medium-high heat just until the mushrooms begin to release some of their liquid.

Spread the tomato sauce over pizza crust and sprinkle the sauce with oregano. Scatter the cooked meat evenly over the sauce. Place turkey ham pieces uniformly over crust. Sprinkle the toppings with basil. Spoon the cooked vegetables uniformly over crust and then add the bell peppers and olives. Top with the cheese. Finally, sprinkle the tarragon over all.

Bake about 30 minutes or until cheese is lightly browned. Remove from the oven and allow the pizza to sit for about 10 minutes before cutting it into 8 wedges with a sharp pizza cutter. Serve two slices to each person.

Nutritional information per serving: 574 calories, 25 grams total fat (9 grams saturated, 6 grams monounsaturated), 40 grams protein, 3 grams fiber, 4 milligrams iron, 94 milligrams cholesterol, 1501 milligrams sodium

NOTE: The high sodium content of this recipe comes from the ham and sausage. If you are trying to reduce sodium in your diet, reduce the amount of ham and sausage and add more ground turkey.

Pecan-Crusted Pork Chops with Orange Sauce and Spiced Pears

These pork chops are crunchy, tangy, and sweet. What else could you possibly want from a main course? Paired with a tossed salad and Spiced Pears, this dish makes an elegant meal for company, for a special occasion, or for no reason at all except the desire for a distinctive dinner.

PECAN-CRUSTED PORK CHOPS WITH ORANGE SAUCE
SERVES 4

1 (11-ounce) can mandarin oranges in light syrup
¼ cup syrup from the mandarin oranges
½ teaspoon ground cinnamon
½ teaspoon ground cumin
Dash cayenne pepper (optional)
½ cup plain nonfat yogurt
1 tablespoon brown mustard
4 garlic cloves, minced
1 teaspoon extra-virgin olive oil
2 tablespoons sweet paprika, divided
½ cup pecans, pieces
½ cup dried breadcrumbs
4 (4-ounce) lean boneless pork chops
1 teaspoon grated orange zest
2 tablespoons freshly squeezed orange juice

Preheat the broiler.

In the container of a blender or food processor, combine the oranges, syrup, cinnamon, cumin, and cayenne pepper, if using. Process until smooth. Pour into a small bowl, cover, and chill.

In medium bowl, combine the yogurt, mustard, garlic, oil, orange juice, and paprika. Set aside. Combine the pecans and bread crumbs in the container of a blender or food processor and process until finely ground. Spread on a plate. Brush each pork chop on both sides with the yogurt mixture; then press into the nut mixture. Broil about six inches from heat on a broiling pan sprayed with nonstick cooking spray, 10 to 15 minutes or until done (no pink remaining), turning carefully halfway through cooking. Use a spatula and try not to dislodge the nut crust when turning.

To serve, drizzle some of the oranges and their sauce on a plate and top with a pork chop.

Nutritional information per serving: 366 calories, 20 grams total fat (4 grams saturated, 10 grams monounsaturated), 27 grams protein, 3 grams fiber, 3 milligrams iron, 67 milligrams cholesterol, 248 milligrams sodium

SPICED PEARS

SERVES 4

2 ripe pears
¼ teaspoon freshly grated nutmeg

Halve the pears and cut out the cores. Slice the pears and divide evenly onto four dessert plates. Sprinkle evenly with the nutmeg and serve immediately.

Nutritional information per serving: 50 calories, 0 gram total fat (0 gram saturated, 0 gram monounsaturated), 0 gram protein, 2 grams fiber, 0 milligram iron, 0 milligram cholesterol, 0 gram sodium

A Better Burger, Baked Fries, and Chopped Salad

Why go out for fast food, with all the associated health risks of such high-fat, high-sodium, and mega-caloric fare, when you can make your own healthier burger and fries at home? This burger has just a little beef, plus chopped mushrooms and onions for flavor. To avoid the risk of mad cow disease, ground beef is allowed in this recipe only if you buy a piece of red muscle meat and grind it yourself at home in a professional quality food processor. Otherwise, you'll have to do without the ground beef and use all ground turkey breast—no cheating! The potatoes are baked instead of fried; and the chopped salad adds color, fiber, vitamins, and a nice crunch.

A BETTER BURGER

SERVES 4

> ½ *pound ground turkey breast*
> ¼ *pound extra-lean ground beef (ground at home, to avoid contamination, from a piece of red muscle meat, or use all ground turkey breast)*
> 1 *slice whole wheat bread, toasted and crumbled into fine crumbs*
> 1 *egg white*
> ½ *cup finely chopped white mushrooms*
> ¼ *cup finely chopped yellow onion*
> 2 *tablespoons low-sodium teriyaki sauce*
> 4 *whole-grain hamburger buns*
> 4 *tomato slices*
> 4 *onion slices*
> 8 *pickle slices*
> 4 *large Romaine lettuce leaves*
> *Condiments: ketchup, mustard, nonfat mayonnaise, to taste*

Preheat the broiler. Spray a broiler pan with nonstick cooking spray.

Put turkey, beef, bread crumbs, egg white, mushrooms, onion, and teriyaki sauce in a large bowl and mix well with your hands. Form into four patties. Place the patties on the unheated rack of a broiler pan.

Broil for 10 minutes 4 inches from heat source, flip hamburgers, and broil for another 5 minutes or until burgers are no longer pink in the middle (use a meat thermometer to ensure the burgers are fully cooked).

Serve on the hamburger buns topped with the tomato, onion, and pickle slices; lettuce; and your favorite condiments.

Nutritional information per serving: 300 calories, 10 grams total fat (3 grams saturated, 3 grams monounsaturated), 23 grams protein, 4 grams fiber, 4 milligrams iron, 55 milligrams cholesterol, 533 milligrams sodium

BAKED FRIES

SERVES 4

2 large or 4 medium baking potatoes
Salt, to taste

Preheat the oven to 400°F. Spray a large baking sheet with nonstick cooking spray.

Cut the potatoes into strips. Arrange them so they aren't touching and spray lightly with cooking spray. Sprinkle lightly with salt. Bake 30 minutes or until the potatoes are tender and lightly browned.

Nutritional information per serving (made with ½ teaspoon salt): 133 calories, 0 gram total fat (0 gram saturated, 0 gram monounsaturated), 3 grams protein, 3 grams fiber, 2 milligrams iron, 0 milligram cholesterol, 303 milligrams sodium

CHOPPED SALAD

SERVES 4

4 cups lettuce leaves, torn into bite-size pieces
2 tomatoes
1 bell pepper
½ small red onion
1 large or 2 medium carrots
½ cucumber, peeled and sliced
1 cup raw broccoli florets

2 ounces low-fat or nonfat Cheddar cheese, shredded
1 tablespoon extra-virgin olive oil
1 tablespoon freshly squeezed lemon juice
2 garlic cloves, minced
1 teaspoon sesame seeds

Chop the lettuce into shreds. Dice the tomatoes, bell pepper, onion, carrots, cucumbers, and broccoli and mix with the lettuce. Sprinkle with the cheese.

In a small bowl, combine the oil, lemon juice, garlic, and sesame seeds. Pour over the salad and toss until thoroughly combined.

Nutritional information per serving: 119 calories, 5 grams total fat (1 gram saturated, 3 grams monounsaturated), 6 grams protein, 4 grams fiber, 1 milligram iron, 3 milligrams cholesterol, 116 milligrams sodium

Shish Kebab Barbecue with Grilled Fruit Skewers

Shish kebabs are fun to make and fun to eat. The variety of meats and veggies on each skewer adds interest and so does the marinated tofu, something beef lovers may not have tried before. Tofu has a cheese-like consistency and takes on the flavor of whatever it is marinated with or cooked with. The grilled fruit skewers are an exotic dessert, perfect for impressing guests. This meal is also perfect for parties. Guests can choose their own meats, vegetables, and fruit combinations.

SHISH KEBAB BARBECUE

SERVES 4

4 ounces firm tofu, cubed
1 tablespoon low-sodium soy sauce
1 garlic clove, chopped or put through a press
1 (4-ounce) chicken breast, cut into four pieces
4 ounces cooked, shelled, deveined jumbo shrimp
1 (4-ounce) piece of lean pork loin, cut into four pieces
1 medium onion, cut into chunks

1 bell pepper, cut into chunks

8 white mushrooms

4 tablespoons good barbecue sauce

Put the tofu, soy sauce, and garlic in a small bowl and allow it to sit for about 30 minutes in the refrigerator.

Cover the grill grate with foil, spray lightly with nonstick cooking spray, and heat the grill according to the manufacturer's instructions.

Thread the ingredients onto four skewers, alternating meat, tofu, and vegetables. Brush with barbecue sauce. Grill, uncovered, until the chicken and pork are cooked through and the vegetables are tender, about 20 minutes. Turn the skewers halfway through the cooking time.

Nutritional information per serving: 205 calories, 8 grams total fat (2 grams saturated, 2 grams monounsaturated), 25 grams protein, 2 grams fiber, 5 milligrams iron, 78 milligrams cholesterol, 342 milligrams sodium

GRILLED FRUIT SKEWERS

SERVES 4

1 medium peach

1 medium apple

1 medium banana

1 medium firm pear

1 medium orange

1 tablespoon freshly squeezed lemon juice

1 teaspoon sugar

¼ teaspoon ground cinnamon

¼ cup nonfat vanilla yogurt

Spray the grate of the grill with nonstick cooking spray. Preheat the grill according to the manufacturer's instructions.

Cut the peach, apple, banana, and pear into eight pieces each. Section the orange. Thread the fruit onto four skewers, alternating the oranges with the other fruits. Brush the fruit with the lemon juice and sprinkle with the sugar and cinnamon. Grill about 10 minutes, until the fruit is heated through, turning halfway through the cooking time. If the fruit is getting soft, you might want to put some foil under it so it doesn't fall through the grill.

To serve, use a fork to slide the warm fruit off the skewers and into bowls. Top each with a spoonful of yogurt.

Nutritional information per serving: 118 calories, 0.5 gram total fat (0 gram saturated, 0 gram monounsaturated), 2 grams protein, 4 grams fiber, 0.3 milligram iron, 0.3 milligram cholesterol, 11 milligrams sodium

Chili Meat Loaf with Homemade Coleslaw

Meat loaf is traditionally made with ground beef; here it takes on a new, lighter, more interesting flavor when made with turkey and pork. You can also make this with half turkey and half extra-lean ground beef—if you're willing to grind your own beef from an extra-lean piece of red muscle meat. The chilies and salsa give this meat loaf a delicious spicy zip. If you serve only four or five people for dinner, you'll have enough meat loaf left-over to make sandwiches the next day. The colorful Homemade Coleslaw is lower in fat, higher in vitamins, and fresher in taste than the kind you buy at the deli.

CHILI MEAT LOAF

SERVES 10

> 2 eggs, beaten
> 1 cup croutons, crushed (put in a sealable bag and roll with a
>   rolling pin, or mash with a masher right in the measuring cup)
>   to one-half crumbs
> ½ yellow onion, chopped
> 1 large celery rib, diced
> 1 4-ounce can (about 3) green chilies, chopped
> 2 garlic cloves, minced
> 1 teaspoon crushed dried basil
> 1 pound ground turkey breast

*1 pound extra-lean ground pork (or extra-lean ground beef, if you
grind your own beef from a piece of extra-lean red muscle
meat)*

1 cup purchased or homemade salsa

Preheat the oven to 350°F.

Combine the eggs, crouton crumbs, onion, celery, chilies, garlic, and basil. Add the ground meats and use your hands to mix until thoroughly combined. Spray a standard 9-inch loaf pan with nonstick cooking spray. Press meat mixture into loaf pan and bake 90 minutes, or until the center is no longer pink and the meat loaf reaches an internal temperature of 170°F.

To serve, carefully pour out any water and/or grease from the bottom of the pan and transfer the meat loaf to a platter. Top with the salsa, slice, and serve.

Nutritional information per serving: 229 calories, 15 grams total fat (5 grams saturated, 0.4 gram monounsaturated), 18 grams protein, 1 gram fiber, 1 milligram iron, 106 milligrams cholesterol, 267 milligrams sodium

HOMEMADE COLESLAW

SERVES 4

½ cup low-fat or nonfat mayonnaise
½ cup plain nonfat yogurt
1 tablespoon cider vinegar
1 teaspoon honey
Dash salt
Dash freshly ground black pepper
2 cups shredded green cabbage
2 cups shredded red cabbage
1 cup shredded carrots
1 cup shredded zucchini
2 celery ribs, minced
½ medium red bell pepper, finely chopped

In a large bowl, combine the mayonnaise, yogurt, vinegar, honey, salt, and black pepper. Mix well. Add the vegetables and mix until thoroughly combined and coated with the dressing. Cover and chill for 2 to 12 hours.

Nutritional information per serving: 35 calories, 0.5 gram total fat (0.1 gram saturated, 0.1 gram monounsaturated), 1 gram protein, 2 grams fiber, 0.4 milligram iron, 1 milligram cholesterol, 240 milligrams sodium

Roasted Tarragon Chicken, Baked Potato, Mixed Greens Salad, and Orange Slices with Cinnamon

This luscious meal is perfect for a Sunday family dinner, a romantic evening for two, or guests. No beef about it!

ROASTED TARRAGON CHICKEN

SERVES 6

> 1 (3-pound) chicken
> 1 small onion, quartered
> 1 celery rib, quartered
> 1 lemon, quartered
> 5 sprigs fresh tarragon, or to taste
> 1 whole lemon
> 1 garlic clove
> 1 tablespoon extra-virgin olive oil
> 1 teaspoon dried tarragon
> Sweet paprika, to taste

Preheat the oven to 375°F.

Remove the giblets from the chicken and discard or set aside for another use. Rinse the chicken inside and out and dry with paper towels. Place the chicken in a roasting pan. Stuff the chicken with the onion, celery, quartered lemon, and 1 sprig of tarragon.

Slice the whole lemon and the garlic as thinly as you can (a sharp serrated knife makes this easier). Loosen the skin over the chicken breast and tuck in the remaining tarragon and the lemon and garlic slices.

Tie the chicken legs together with twine, tuck the wings back and under the chicken, and tuck in or skewer the neck skin closed. Brush the skin with the oil; then sprinkle with the dried tarragon and paprika.

Bake about 1 hour or until the thigh temperature reaches 180° to 185°F, the thigh bone moves easily, and the juices run clear when the skin is pricked with a fork. Remove the chicken from the oven and allow it to sit for 15 minutes. Slice the chicken, removing and discarding skin, tarragon, lemon, and garlic beneath the skin as you go. Serve 3 to 4 ounces of chicken per person.

Nutritional information per serving: 119 calories, 10 grams total fat (2 grams saturated, 5 grams monounsaturated), 4 grams protein, 1 gram fiber, 1 milligram iron, 15 milligrams cholesterol, 19 milligrams sodium

BAKED POTATO

SERVES 6

6 baking potatoes
6 teaspoons low-fat or nonfat sour cream

Preheat oven to 400°F. Scrub potatoes with a brush and prick all over with a fork. Place in preheated oven directly on the rack and bake for one hour. You can also bake them right along with the chicken, above. Just put them on the lower oven rack. They should be done at about the same time. To serve, slice each potato and top each with 1 teaspoon of sour cream.

Nutritional information per serving: 139 calories, 0 gram total fat (0 gram saturated, 0 gram monounsaturated), 3 grams protein, 3 grams fiber, 2 milligrams iron, 0 milligram cholesterol, 14 milligrams sodium

MIXED GREENS SALAD

SERVES 6

> *12 cups mixed greens, such as head lettuce, leaf lettuce, spinach,*
> *kale, arugula, endive, radicchio, Romaine, Swiss chard,*
> *watercress, and cabbage*
> *6 tablespoons low-fat dressing*

Tear the greens into bite-size pieces. Serve 2 cups and 1 tablespoon of dressing per person.

Nutritional information per serving of salad side dish: 42 calories, 2 grams total fat (0.4 gram saturated, 0.5 gram monounsaturated), 2 grams protein, 2 grams fiber, 1 milligram iron, 0 milligram cholesterol, 181 milligrams sodium

ORANGE SLICES WITH CINNAMON

SERVES 6

> *3 teaspoons sugar*
> *1 ½ teaspoons ground cinnamon*
> *6 medium oranges or tangerines*

Mix the sugar and cinnamon together in a small bowl. Peel and quarter the oranges and remove the pith and any seeds. Divide the oranges evenly among six dessert bowls, topping each evenly with the sugar and cinnamon mix.

Nutritional information per serving: 47 calories, 0 gram total fat (0 gram saturated, 0 gram monounsaturated), 1 gram protein, 2 grams fiber, 0 milligram iron, 0 milligram cholesterol, 1 milligram sodium

Turkey Sausage Subs and Banana Wheels with Milk and Honey

The next time you think you want a cheeseburger and fries, try this hearty recipe instead. You'll feel much better afterward. These sub sandwiches are big and filling but contain a lot less fat than a typical sausage sub. The vegetables add fiber and nutrients as well as flavor, and the Banana Wheels with Milk and Honey will have your insides humming with quiet satisfaction.

Be sure the turkey sausage you use in this recipe is 100 percent beef-free, including the casings, and preferably organic. Talk to your butcher, and if you buy from the meat case, remember that you can't necessarily trust the label. Health food markets and other sources of organic, free-range meats may be more likely to have sausages that are trustworthy. Many companies now specialize in products that use only organic meat without hormones and antibiotics, and their sausages are likely to contain only turkey, sea salt, and spices, or other combinations of low-fat, non-beef ingredients. If the sausage is made in the store, ask if the grinders being used ever grind beef. Increasingly, food sellers are becoming aware of the dangers of and/or public concern about beef and are more likely to take precautions.

TURKEY SAUSAGE SUBS

SERVES 4

> 4 whole wheat sub rolls
> 12 ounces low-fat, low-sodium 100 percent turkey sausage, or other non-beef sausage, such as chicken or seafood or even meatless, thinly sliced
> 8 ounces part skim Mozzarella cheese, sliced
> 1 medium bell pepper, sliced into strips
> 1 medium onion, sliced into strips
> 4 large mushrooms, sliced
> 1½ teaspoons chili powder
> Brown mustard, to taste (optional)

Spray a large nonstick skillet and heat over medium heat. Add the sausage, bell pepper, onion, mushrooms, and chili powder. Cook, stirring, until the vegetables are tender, about 10 minutes.

Preheat broiler or toaster oven.

Slice the rolls and toast them until just warm and slightly browned. Watch them carefully so they don't burn. If you'd like, spread brown mustard on the rolls. Spoon the sausage and vegetables evenly on the rolls. Top each with cheese slices. Return to the broiler for 1 minute, or even less, just long enough to melt the cheese.

Nutritional information per serving: 637 calories, 30 grams total fat (15 grams saturated, 0.3 gram monounsaturated), 38 grams protein, 6 grams fiber, 12 milligrams iron, 82 milligrams cholesterol, 1416 milligrams sodium

NOTE: To reduce the sodium, use low-sodium cheese and choose the lowest-sodium brands of beef-free sausage you can find.

BANANA WHEELS WITH MILK AND HONEY

SERVES 4

> *4 medium ripe bananas*
> *2 cups low-fat milk*
> *4 tablespoons honey*
> *¼ teaspoon freshly grated nutmeg or ground cinnamon*

Slice the bananas into wheels and divide among four dessert bowls. Heat the milk in a medium saucepan over medium heat or in the microwave for about two minutes on high just until warm, not scalded. Pour evenly in each bowl of fruit. Drizzle each with 1 tablespoon honey, and sprinkle on a pinch of nutmeg.

Nutritional information per serving: 133 calories, 2 grams total fat (0.8 gram saturated, 0.3 gram monounsaturated), 5 grams protein, 2 grams fiber, 0 milligram iron, 8 milligrams cholesterol, 73 milligrams sodium

MONITOR YOUR PROGRESS—STEP 2

❑ I am choosing very lean meats, such as skinless white-meat chicken or turkey, on most days of the week.

❑ I am incorporating fish sources of omega-3 fatty acids into my diet at least once a week.

❑ I am reducing the number of days each week I include beef in my meal plans.

❑ I am limiting my beef portions to 3 ounces.

❑ I am choosing ground turkey or chicken exclusively, instead of using any ground beef—even home ground—in meal preparation.

❑ I am confirming with the local butcher or directly with the manu-facturer that the turkey sausage I buy, or any kind of sausage I cook with, does not contain any added beef or beef by-products.

Once you've mastered step 2, proceed to step 3.

15

Recipes
Step 3: Incorporate

The key concept for step 3 is *incorporate.* The nutritional advice and recipes in this chapter provide you with the reasons and how-to for incorporating more plant foods into your diet. The less beef (and meat in general) you eat, the more you'll need to fill your diet with something else; and unless that something else is healthy, hearty, and satisfying, you probably won't be able to stick with a beef-free diet. But plant foods can fit the bill. When whole grains, vegetables, fruits, legumes, nuts, and seeds form the basis of your diet, you're eating the way your body was designed to eat.

Most people are probably familiar with the U.S. Department of Agriculture's (USDA) food pyramid, and possibly other food pyramids as well, such as the Mediterranean Diet pyramid. In the food pyramids for most healthy eating plans, the bottom tier—the largest tier of all, the one on which all the other food groups rest—is the grains group. On top of that are fruits and vegetables. In other words, most of the food we eat should come from plants. (For a look at the USDA Food Pyramid, see Chapter 8.)

Eating plant foods goes beyond the notion of just "eat your vegetables." For most of us, this familiar phrase was almost a daily dinnertime recital from our parents or guardians. Indeed, we came to identify vegetables as "nutritious," sources of vitamins and minerals. But the glob of green stuff that was commonly served up to Americans during the

1950s through the 1970s was often anything but appetizing; thus we came to associate the idea of "nutritious food" with something really awful.

But American culinary trends have changed. Vegetables and other plant foods are more likely to be prepared in fresh, exciting ways, full of texture, color, and flavor. Our culinary horizons are broadening, becoming more international, more natural, and more likely to emphasize plant foods over meat and dairy. Vegetables, fruits, and grains are likely to be steamed, sautéed, grilled, broiled, poached, or simmered in tasty broth with seasonings and flavorings never imagined in the 1950s kitchen. No longer merely mandatory side dishes, plant foods have truly come into their own.

And today, vegetables are not considered as just a source of vitamins and minerals (although this is certainly a good reason to eat your vegetables!). Plant foods of all kinds—whole grains, legumes, nuts, seeds, vegetables, and fruits—have also been found to be powerful fighters of chronic diseases, providing us with the ammunition to help protect the health of our bodies as well as of our minds.

Some experts believe that up to 70 percent of cancers may be related to diet. Although genetics and other lifestyle choices, such as smoking, certainly influence the rates of chronic diseases, evidence suggests that simple dietary changes—changes anyone can implement—can make a real difference in lowering the risk of developing certain cancers. All you need to do is add more delicious plant foods into your regular meals.

One reason plant foods help us in our fight against chronic diseases, such as cancer and heart disease, and help us increase our longevity is they are rich in antioxidants. Antioxidants are powerful substances that combat the negative onslaught of free radicals that invade our bodies from, among other things, the polluted air we breathe. Antioxidants include vitamins C, E, and A (in the form of beta-carotene), and minerals such as selenium. The evidence of the effectiveness of these antioxidants when taken in supplement form, however, is controversial. Some studies show that supplements can offer some cancer protection. Other studies refute this claim, and one study even suggests that beta-carotene supplements could actually increase the risk of cancer in smokers. But when it comes to antioxidants in the natural plant foods we eat, the news is all good. Ingesting antioxidant vitamins, minerals, or phytochemicals (see below) in their natural form helps the human body strengthen its immune system and combat certain physiological reactions that could contribute to the development of cancer, heart disease, and many other age-associated disorders. Foods rich in antioxidants include citrus fruits; leafy greens; and any vegetable or fruit with a deep orange or yellow color, like cantaloupes, carrots, mangoes, sweet potatoes, and peaches.

Another exciting and recently discovered reason plant foods are so beneficial to our health is that they are rich sources of phytochemicals. *Phytochemical* means plant (*phtyo-*) chemicals, and some phytochemicals are antioxidants. As the name implies, they are only found in plant foods, not in animal foods (such as beef). Phytochemicals are nonvitamin, nonmineral substances found to be beneficial to our health in several ways. From slowing the aging process to strengthening our immune systems to preventing and maybe even *reversing* the onslaught of cancer and other chronic diseases, these substances are indeed the "new age of nutrition" (as this field of research has been dubbed) and something we will certainly be hearing more about. Scientists suspect thousands of phytochemicals exist, although they have isolated only a few. Here are some that we know about already:

- *Lycopene:* found in red fruits and vegetables (such as tomatoes and watermelon); thought to reduce the risk of certain cancers (such as prostate cancer).
- *Allium compounds:* found in onions and garlic; thought to decrease blood pressure, cholesterol levels, and the blood's tendency to clot; may also fight cancer.
- *Flavonoids:* include quercetin, found in tea, wine, and onions;

isoflavones, found in soybeans; and catechins, found in green tea; thought to have antifungal properties, may lower cholesterol, and seem to have an anticancer effect.

■ *Lutein and zeaxanthin:* found in spinach; thought to protect the eyes from the degenerative effects of aging.

When fat is found in plant foods (most plant foods are virtually fat free!), it is likely to be in the form of heart-healthy monounsaturated fat and/or omega-3 fatty acids. This is another reason why plant foods are so beneficial to our health. Plant foods are also the only source of fiber—thus something you won't get in meat and dairy products—that is essential to keep the digestive system running smoothly. Diets rich in fiber are also linked to reduced rates of digestive cancers (like colon and stomach cancer) and heart disease.

Adding plant foods can be a lot more fun than putting some lettuce in a salad bowl next to your plate of meat. Plant foods can infuse every part of the meal, adding color, texture, flavor, and freshness to any dish. Plant foods are filling, satisfying, and rewarding to eat. You feel so good afterward that you won't believe you are sacrificing a thing . . . and you aren't! The recipes given in this chapter will give you some great ideas for putting more plant foods, and more life, into your meals. Several recipes include side-dish options, others are filling, well-rounded stand-alone meals that contain all the nutrients you need.

RECIPES

LENTIL STEW WITH HAM

Lentils are a nutrient-packed legume that has the texture of meat without any of the fat or cholesterol. Ounce for ounce, lentils have the same amount of protein as lean ground beef—without the potential health risk of mad cow disease or danger of bacterial contamination from E. coli. Flavor the lentils with fresh vegetables, smoky cumin, and just a bit of turkey ham for a satisfying main-course stew. Add a quality, whole-grain bread from the bakery and a salad of leafy greens and nonfat dressing for a simple, elegant, and nutritious dinner.

SERVES 4

> 1 tablespoon extra-virgin olive oil
> 1 medium carrot, diced
> 1 celery rib, diced
> 1 medium yellow onion, chopped
> 1 garlic clove, minced or put through a press
> 2 ounces lean turkey ham, diced
> 4 cups plus 2 tablespoons beef broth (or substitute chicken or
>   vegetable broth, or water)
> 1 cup lentils
> 1 teaspoon ground cumin
> 1 teaspoon salt
> Pinch hot red pepper flakes
> 1 tablespoon sweet sherry (optional)

Heat the oil in a Dutch oven over medium-high heat. Add the carrot, celery, onion, garlic, turkey ham, and 2 tablespoons of the beef broth. Cook, stirring, until the vegetables are just tender.

Add the remaining ingredients. Bring to a boil; then reduce the heat. Simmer the stew uncovered for 1 hour or until lentils are tender and flavors are combined, adding a small amount of water or broth if it gets too dry. Skim off any foam and serve with thick slices of whole-grain bread and a green salad.

Nutritional information per serving: 285 calories, 8 grams total fat (1 gram saturated, 3 grams monounsaturated), 23 grams protein, 16 grams fiber, 5 milligrams iron, 12 milligrams cholesterol, 2431 milligrams sodium

NOTE: To reduce the sodium in this recipe, use reduced-sodium broth, or use water instead of broth. The real significant source of sodium in this recipe is the turkey ham; you may also reduce the amount of turkey ham used and this will help cut sodium content.

CHEESY RICE CASSEROLE

This satisfying main course is comfort food with just a little of the meat and fat. Most of what makes this casserole filling are grains, beans, and vegetables. Cheesy Rice Casserole is delicious with a crisp salad or served all by itself. It contains everything you need for a well-rounded meal.

SERVES 4

> 1 tablespoon canola oil
> 1 medium onion, chopped
> 2 garlic cloves, minced or put through a press
> ½ medium bell pepper, chopped
> 1 medium carrot, grated
> 1 celery rib, diced
> ½ cup sliced white mushrooms
> 2 cups cooked brown rice
> 1 (4-ounce) can chopped green chilies, or 3 chilies, diced
> 4 ounces Neufchâtel cheese or low-fat or nonfat cream cheese, at
>   room temperature
> ½ teaspoon crushed dried basil
> 2 ounces cooked white-meat chicken, finely chopped
> 4 ounces low-fat Cheddar cheese, shredded

Preheat the oven to 375°F.

Heat the oil in a large skillet over medium-high heat. Add the onion, garlic, bell pepper, carrot, celery, and mushrooms, and cook, stirring occasionally, until tender, about 8 minutes.

In a large bowl, combine the rice, green chilies, Neufchâtel cheese, basil, and chicken. Add the onion mixture and stir to combine. Spoon into a 1-quart casserole (ungreased) and bake uncovered 30 minutes, or until casserole is heated through. Remove from the oven and immediately sprinkle with the Cheddar cheese. Let the casserole sit 10 minutes; then serve.

Nutritional information per serving: 327 calories, 14 grams total fat (6 grams saturated, 5 grams monounsaturated), 18 grams protein, 5 grams fiber, 1 milligram iron, 39 milligrams cholesterol, 422 milligrams sodium

HEALTHIER HASH

Hash has always been a frugal dish, but when the potatoes, vegetables, and meat are fried in generous portions of fat, the nutritional benefit of all those plant foods is easily overcome by the nutritional disaster of all that fat. This version uses just enough fat for flavor, but allows the vegetables to shine. A salad and some fresh fruit for dessert are the only necessary complements.

SERVES 4

> *1 tablespoon extra-virgin olive oil*
> *1 medium onion, chopped*
> *3 medium potatoes, boiled and diced*
> *2 cups diced root vegetables*
> *4 ounces minced turkey ham*

Warm the oil in a large nonstick skillet over medium-high heat. Add the remaining ingredients, cooking and stirring just until combined. Reduce heat to medium-low. Then, press the mixture down with a spatula to compress it. Let it cook, without stirring, until heated through, about 15 minutes. Slide the hash onto a plate and cut it into quarters to serve.

Nutritional information per serving: 197 calories, 5 grams total fat (1 gram saturated, 4 grams monounsaturated), 9 grams protein, 6 grams fiber, 2 milligrams iron, 19 milligrams cholesterol, 291 milligrams sodium

NOTE: Use whatever root vegetables you like, including boiled turnips, parsnips, kohlrabi, beets, or raw carrots.

Fiesta Stuffed Peppers and Homemade Custard with Fruit

These spicy, colorful peppers are exciting and fun to eat, as well as being high in protein, fiber, vitamins, and minerals. Accompanied by smooth, cool homemade custard with fruit for dessert, this meal will take your palate through a range of taste sensations, leaving you feeling supremely satisfied afterward.

FIESTA STUFFED PEPPERS

SERVES 4

> *4 large red bell peppers*
> *½ pound ground turkey breast*
> *1 medium onion*
> *1 cup cooked yellow rice (the packaged yellow rice available in most grocery stores that has saffron and spices already added works best; just cook according to package directions)*
> *½ cup canned black beans, rinsed and drained*
> *1 (4-ounce) can chopped green chilies*
> *1 tablespoon chili powder*
> *4 ounces nonfat Cheddar cheese, shredded*
> *2 cups purchased salsa, at room temperature*

Preheat the oven to 400°F. Cut the tops off the bell peppers and remove seeds and ribs. Arrange them in a square baking pan.

Heat a large skillet over medium heat. Cook the ground turkey until browned; drain. Add the onion, rice, beans, green chilies, and chili powder. Cook and stir until combined and heated through, about 10 minutes. Add the cheese and mix until combined.

Spoon the turkey mixture into the bell pepper shells. (If you have extra filling, save it to eat on its own the next day.) Bake 15 minutes, or until heated through. Remove from the oven and top the stuffed peppers with salsa. Serve in bowls.

Nutritional information per serving: 306 calories, 6 grams total fat (1 gram saturated, 2 grams monounsaturated), 22 grams protein, 1 gram fiber, 3 milligrams iron, 48 milligrams cholesterol, 1418 milligrams sodium

NOTE: To cut sodium in this recipe, use low-sodium cheese, and make sure the black beans are thoroughly rinsed. Using white or brown rice instead of packaged yellow rice will also reduce sodium, but the flavor will be different.

HOMEMADE CUSTARD WITH FRUIT

SERVES 4

> *3 eggs*
> *1½ cups low-fat or nonfat milk*
> *⅓ cup plus 1 tablespoon packed brown sugar*
> *Boiling water, for baking*
> *Ground cinnamon, to taste*
> *½ cup fresh or frozen strawberries, blueberries, raspberries, blackberries, or cherries*

Preheat the oven to 325°F.

In a medium bowl, beat the eggs with a fork. Add the milk and sugar. Beat with a fork until just combined but not foamy. Pour into four custard cups. Place the custard cups in a baking pan. Sprinkle each with a dash of cinnamon.

Put the baking pan onto the oven rack; then carefully pour boiling water into the baking pan until it comes almost halfway up the sides of the custard cups. Be careful not to splash water into the custard. (Using a tea kettle makes this job easier.) Bake 30 to 45 minutes, or until a knife inserted into one of the custards comes out clean. Remove the custard cups from the water and cool on a rack about 10 minutes before serving or cool, chill, and serve cold in the custard cups (no need to unmold, unless you want to). Top each custard cup with one-quarter of the fruit.

Nutritional information per serving: 193 calories, 5 grams total fat (2 grams saturated, 2 grams monounsaturated), 8 grams protein, 1 gram fiber, 1 milligram iron, 165 milligrams cholesterol, 105 milligrams sodium

PEPPER STIR-FRY

Pepper beef is an old standard in Chinese restaurants and stir-fry cookbooks. Our version—which uses just a little beef along with shrimp, marinated tofu, and lots of juicy peppers—is better because it calls for cooking the meat and vegetables in broth rather than in oil. It may not taste exactly like stir-fry, but it has an equally interesting flavor. If you still aren't sure about tofu, try it in this recipe where it blends effortlessly with the beef and shrimp. C'mon. We dare you to try it! Plums make a simple, elegant finish to this filling dinner.

SERVES 4

> *1 cup brown or white rice, uncooked*
> *3 tablespoons Worcestershire sauce*
> *3 tablespoons soy sauce*
> *¼ cup dry white wine or fresh orange juice*
> *1 teaspoon ground ginger*
> *1 teaspoon sugar*
> *¼ teaspoon hot red pepper flakes (optional)*
> *1 tablespoon cornstarch*
> *4 ounces firm tofu, diced*
> *1 cup beef broth (or substitute chicken or vegetable broth, or water)*
> *2 ounces lean beef cut into thin slices*
> *2 green bell peppers, sliced into rings*
> *2 red bell peppers, sliced into rings*
> *1 large carrot, sliced on the bias*
> *1 medium onion, chopped*
> *2 garlic cloves, minced or put through a press*
> *4 ounces fresh raw shrimp, shelled, tails removed*

Cook the rice according to the package's directions.

While the rice is cooking, combine the Worcestershire sauce, soy sauce, wine, ginger, sugar, and red pepper in a medium bowl. Using a fork, whisk in the cornstarch until smooth. Gently mix in the tofu and set aside.

Heat 1 cup of the beef broth in a large skillet over medium-high heat. Add the beef and cook until it turns brown, about 5 minutes. Add the bell peppers, carrot, onion, and garlic. Lower the heat and simmer until the vegetables are tender, about 10 minutes. Add the shrimp and cook until it turns pink, about 5 minutes.

Remove the tofu cubes from the marinade with a slotted spoon and add it to the skillet. Pour the marinade over the entire mixture and cook, stirring, until thickened into a sauce-like consistency, 10 to 15 minutes. Serve over the hot rice.

Nutritional information per serving: 349 calories, 5 grams total fat (1 gram saturated, 1 gram monounsaturated), 20 grams protein, 6 grams fiber, 4 milligrams iron, 52 milligrams cholesterol, 1475 milligrams sodium

NOTE: To reduce the sodium in this recipe, use reduced-sodium soy sauce, Worcestershire sauce, and broth.

Pasta Casserole with Chicken and White Beans and Low-Fat Carrot-Walnut Bread

This grown-up version of macaroni and cheese is lower in fat than the childhood dish you remember. But it still ranks high on the comfort-food scale. Flavored with chicken and white beans, this casserole is a main course. A salad and nutritious carrot and nut bread round out the meal.

PASTA CASSEROLE WITH CHICKEN AND WHITE BEANS

SERVES 4

> *8 ounces dried stubby pasta, such as elbow macaroni, ziti, or wagon wheels*
> *4 ounces chicken breast, diced*
> *1 teaspoon chili powder*
> *1 (15-ounce) can white beans, drained and rinsed*
> *½ cup low-fat ricotta cheese*

½ cup low-fat cottage cheese
½ cup low-fat or nonfat milk
1 cup canned or fresh diced tomatoes
1 teaspoon crushed dried basil
½ teaspoon garlic powder
Dash salt
Dash freshly ground black pepper
4 ounces low-fat or nonfat Cheddar cheese, shredded

Preheat the oven to 350°F.

Cook the pasta according to the package's directions until tender but not overdone. Drain and set aside.

Spray a small skillet with nonstick cooking spray and heat over medium-high heat. Cook the chicken and chili powder until the chicken is cooked through, about 15 minutes.

In a large bowl, combine the chicken and chili mixture, beans, ricotta cheese, cottage cheese, milk, tomatoes, basil, garlic powder, salt, and pepper. Add the pasta and toss to coat. Spoon into an ungreased casserole and bake, uncovered, 30 minutes. Remove from the oven and sprinkle with the Cheddar cheese. Return to the oven and bake about 15 minutes more, or until the Cheddar is melted. Serve in bowls with a green salad on the side.

Nutritional information per serving: 513 calories, 7 grams total fat (3 grams saturated, 0 gram monounsaturated), 37 grams protein, 8 grams fiber, 3 milligrams iron, 35 milligrams cholesterol, 820 milligrams sodium

LOW-FAT CARROT-WALNUT BREAD

SERVES 18

2 cups all-purpose flour
½ cup wheat germ
1½ cups packed brown sugar
2 teaspoons baking powder
1 teaspoon baking soda
½ teaspoon salt

1 teaspoon ground cinnamon

½ teaspoon freshly ground nutmeg

¼ cup extra-virgin olive oil

1 egg

1 cup unsweetened applesauce

1 (11-ounce) can mandarin oranges in light syrup, drained

1 cup grated carrots

2 ounces chopped walnuts

1 teaspoon vanilla extract

Preheat the oven to 350°F. Spray an 8-inch loaf pan lightly with nonstick cooking spray.

In a large bowl, combine the flour, wheat germ, sugar, baking powder, baking soda, salt, cinnamon, and nutmeg. Add the remaining ingredients and mix lightly with a fork until combined.

Pour into the prepared pan and bake 1 hour, or until a toothpick inserted in the middle comes out clean. Cool before slicing.

Nutritional information per serving: 195 calories, 5 grams total fat (1 gram saturated, 3 grams monounsaturated), 3 grams protein, 1 gram fiber, 2 milligrams iron, 10 milligrams cholesterol, 158 milligrams sodium

Red Beans and Rice and Spicy Corn Muffins

This meal combines high-protein grains and legumes with the spiciness of classic Cajun fare for a traditional Southern meal done over with less fat . . . but no less flavor. A note about the ingredients in this dish: You can make this dish even more economically if you start with dried beans—as is the conventional method—but these days, time is limited for many of us, and canned beans seem so much easier. Canned beans aren't exactly expensive, either. They certainly make this dish a snap to whip up when the mood strikes; and as long as you rinse off all the extra salt, canned beans are just as nutritious as the dried.

RED BEANS AND RICE

SERVES 4

> 2 (15-ounce) cans red beans, rinsed, and drained well (see Note)
> ½ cup beef broth (or substitute chicken or vegetable broth,
>   or water)
> 1 medium onion, finely chopped
> 2 celery ribs, finely chopped
> 1 green bell pepper, finely chopped
> 1 (4-ounce) can whole green chilies, finely chopped (about 3 chilies)
> 2 garlic cloves, minced or put through press
> 2 bay leaves
> 1 teaspoon crushed dried thyme
> ½ teaspoon freshly ground black pepper
> ½ teaspoon cayenne pepper, or to taste
> 2 ounces turkey ham, finely chopped
> 2 ounces low-fat turkey sausage, thinly sliced
> 2 cups cooked rice, hot

Combine all the ingredients in a large saucepan and heat over medium-low heat until simmering. Allow to simmer about 30 minutes. To serve, ladle over the rice.

Nutritional information per serving: 91 calories, 4 grams total fat (1 gram saturated, 1 gram monounsaturated), 7 grams protein, 2 grams fiber, 1 milligram iron, 33 milligrams cholesterol, 596 milligrams sodium

NOTE: If you can't find a can labeled "red beans," use pinto beans, pink beans, chili beans, or light red kidney beans.

SPICY CORN MUFFINS

These are so good, you may have trouble stopping at just one!

SERVES 12

> 1 cup cornmeal
> 1 cup unbleached white flour
> 2 teaspoons baking powder

½ teaspoon baking soda

½ teaspoon salt

1 cup buttermilk or plain nonfat yogurt

2 eggs, lightly beaten

1 cup fresh corn kernels or canned and drained kernels or frozen
*   and thawed kernels*

1 (4-ounce) can chopped green chilies

Sweet paprika, for garnish

Preheat the oven to 400°F. Spray a 12-cup medium muffin tin with nonstick cooking spray.

In a large bowl, mix the cornmeal, flour, baking powder, baking soda, and salt until well combined. Add the buttermilk, eggs, corn kernels, and chilies. Mix with a fork just until combined. Don't over mix.

Spoon evenly into the muffin tin and sprinkle each cup with a little paprika. Bake 15 minutes, or until the muffins turn golden brown. Allow to cool, slightly, on a rack. Serve warm.

Nutritional information per serving: 114 calories, 2 grams total fat (0.4 gram saturated, 0.5 gram monounsaturated), 1 gram protein, 1 gram fiber, 1 milligram iron, 32 milligrams cholesterol, 253 milligrams sodium

SALMON STEW

This dish is so delicious that you won't mind sacrificing a perfectly good salmon filet to the soup pot. A crunchy breadstick purchased from the bakery is all this hearty stew needs in the way of accompaniment.

Serves 4

1 tablespoon extra-virgin olive oil

1 medium onion, chopped

4 celery ribs, chopped

2 garlic cloves, chopped

1 pound fresh mushrooms, sliced

1 cup canned diced tomatoes

2 cups low-fat chicken broth

1 teaspoon dried oregano

1 teaspoon hot red pepper flakes

1 (12-ounce) salmon filet, skin removed, cut into chunks

2 tablespoons chopped fresh cilantro

Heat the oil over medium heat in a nonstick saucepan. Add the onion, celery, garlic, and mushrooms, and sauté until tender, about 5 minutes. Add the tomatoes, broth, oregano, and red pepper flakes. Increase the heat to medium-high and bring the stew to a boil. Add the salmon and reduce the heat. Simmer until the salmon is cooked through, about 10 minutes more. Remove from the heat and stir in the cilantro.

To serve, ladle into bowls. Pass fresh breadsticks from the bakery.

Nutritional information per serving: 260 calories, 11 grams total fat (2 grams saturated, 5 grams monounsaturated), 27 grams protein, 4 grams fiber, 3 milligrams iron, 48 milligrams cholesterol, 945 milligrams sodium

Chicken Pot Pies and Homemade Applesauce

These pot pies aren't really pot pies in the traditional sense, which are usually surrounded or topped with pie crust or biscuit dough. These pot pies are topped with crisp baked tortilla wedges . . . perfect for dipping. Add a salad on the side and serve the easy applesauce for dessert, and your meal is complete.

CHICKEN POT PIES

SERVES 4

2 corn tortillas, about 6 inches in diameter

2 cups chicken broth

12 ounces chicken breast, chopped

1 medium onion, chopped

2 garlic cloves, minced or put through a press

1 cup canned white beans, rinsed, drained, and mashed with a fork

1 medium carrot, diced

2 celery ribs, diced

*½ cup fresh peas or canned and drained peas or frozen and thawed
    peas*

½ teaspoon crushed dried sage

⅛ teaspoon ground cloves

½ cup low-fat or nonfat milk

Preheat the oven to 400°F.

Spray the tortillas on both sides with nonstick cooking spray. Cut
each tortilla into 16 wedges with a pizza cutter. Place on a baking sheet
and bake about 10 minutes, until just crisp but not yet brown.

Reduce the oven temperature to 350°F.

Put the chicken broth and chicken in a medium saucepan. Bring to
a boil and poach the chicken until cooked through and broth is
reduced by half, about 20 minutes. Add the onions, garlic, beans, carrots, celery, peas, sage, and cloves. Simmer, stirring occasionally, until
the vegetables are tender, about 15 minutes more. If the mixture gets
too dry, add a bit of water or more chicken broth, but just 1 tablespoon
at a time. The mixture shouldn't be soupy. Stir in the milk and remove
from the heat.

Ladle the mixture into four ovenproof individual casserole dishes.
Top each with eight tortilla wedges arranged to cover the surface. Bake
the pot pies about 25 minutes, or until hot and bubbly. Serve warm.

Nutritional information per serving: 329 calories, 9 grams total fat (2 grams saturated, 1 gram
monounsaturated), 38 grams protein, 6 grams fiber, 3 milligrams iron, 73 milligrams cholesterol,
1149 milligrams sodium

NOTE: To reduce sodium, use low-sodium chicken broth and be sure
the canned beans are well rinsed and drained.

HOMEMADE APPLESAUCE

SERVES 4

> 5 medium cooking apples, like Granny Smith, peeled, cored, and cut
> into quarters
> ¾ cup apple juice
> ¼ cup packed brown sugar
> ¼ teaspoon ground cinnamon

In a large saucepan or Dutch oven, combine all the ingredients. Bring to a boil, reduce the heat, and simmer 10 minutes. Remove from the heat and mash the mixture by hand for a coarse texture or process in a blender for a smooth texture. Cool and refrigerate, covered, for about 2 hours. Serve chilled.

Nutritional information per serving: 174 calories, 0 gram total fat (0 gram saturated, 0 gram monounsaturated), 0 gram protein, 6 grams fiber, 1 milligram iron, 0 milligram cholesterol, 7 milligrams sodium

Seaside Salad and Tropical Fruit Salad

The light seafood salad is essentially tuna salad with pasta. Chilled, it's perfect for summer, especially when served with the fruit salad. After eating this meal for lunch, you'll feel light, full of energy, and ready to hit the beach.

SEASIDE SALAD

SERVES 4

> 2 cups uncooked shell-shaped pasta
> 2 (9-ounce) cans tuna packed in water, drained
> 2 medium carrots, cut into peels with a vegetable peeler
> 2 celery ribs, chopped
> ½ medium cucumber, peeled, quartered, and sliced
> 1 medium tomato, seeded and chopped

2 teaspoons dried dill or 4 teaspoons fresh

4 tablespoons low-fat mayonnaise

Cook the pasta according to the package's directions. Drain and allow to cool to about room temperature (rinsing with cold water should do the trick).

In a large bowl, combine the pasta with the remaining ingredients. Toss to coat. Cover and refrigerate for 1 to 12 hours. Serve with the Tropical Fruit Salad.

Nutritional information per serving: 350 calories, 3 grams total fat (0.5 gram saturated, 0.4 gram monounsaturated), 29 grams protein, 4 grams fiber, 3 milligrams iron, 25 milligrams cholesterol, 455 milligrams sodium

TROPICAL FRUIT SALAD

SERVES 4

1 cup fresh or canned pineapple cubes, drained

1 (11-ounce) can mandarin oranges in light syrup, drained

½ medium cantaloupe, cubed

4 kiwis, halved, and sliced

1 medium banana, sliced

1 teaspoon freshly squeezed lemon juice

1 tablespoon pineapple juice

1 tablespoon orange blossom honey

In a large bowl, combine the fruit. Sprinkle with the lemon and pineapple juices. Toss gently to coat. Drizzle with the honey. Serve immediately.

Nutritional information per serving: 184 calories, 1 gram total fat (0.1 gram saturated, 0.1 gram monounsaturated), 2 grams protein, 5 grams fiber, 1 milligram iron, 0 milligram cholesterol, 22 milligrams sodium

MONITOR YOUR PROGRESS—STEP 3

❑ I am incorporating vegetables into at least one of my meals per day.

❑ I am incorporating fruits (fresh, canned, or frozen fruits or pure fruit juice) into my meals at least once a day.

❑ I am incorporating whole grains (like whole grain bread) into my meals at least once a day.

❑ I am incorporating legumes into my meals at least once a week.

❑ I am including nuts or seeds in my meals at least once a week.

❑ I am incorporating fish sources of omega-3 fatty acids into my diet at least once a week.

❑ I have reduced the number of meals that include beef in my diet to no more than one every two weeks.

❑ I am limiting my beef portions to 3 ounces.

Once you've mastered step 3, proceed to step 4—the final Beef Buster step!

16

Recipes
Step 4: Eliminate

Congratulations! You've made it to the last step in the Beef Busters process. You can feel reassured that by following the steps and guidelines given in this book, you have chosen a dietary lifestyle that is healthy and beneficial and will help you stave off many chronic diseases, increasing your chances for a long, healthy life. But you have one more step to go; and the key concept for step 4 is *eliminate*. In this step, you will take that last leap in the direction you've been heading all along. You'll eliminate beef completely from your diet.

You are already comfortable with replacing beef with other leaner cuts of meat and fish. When you need to satisfy an occasional craving for ground beef, you are choosing an extra-lean cut of red muscle meat to grind your own beef at home. You are avoiding processed foods, such as prepared spaghetti sauces with ground meat. And you are avoiding any sausage or hot-dog product that contains a mixture of beef or beef by-products. Of course, ground turkey and ground chicken can cure your craving, and many people find ground soy products equally satisfying. You are already comfortable with adding more plant foods to your diet. By now, giving up beef may seem easy. Maybe you've already accomplished this step without thinking much about it. That's great! Studies show that populations that eat a primarily plant-based diet and only small to moderate amounts of meat (usually fish and poultry) have traditionally had very low rates of chronic disease such as heart disease, cancer, diabetes, osteoporosis, obesity . . . the list goes on. These groups, such as people living in the Mediterranean region, have a reputation for living long lives and maintaining remarkable mental health, even in old age.

Let's look back at what you've accomplished so far. In step 1, *reduce*, you cut down not only your portion sizes of beef and the number of times you ate beef each week but the amount of bad-for-your-heart saturated fat you ate by switching to leaner cuts of beef. You learned to grind your own ground beef at home and to avoid sausage products containing beef, or processed foods that include ground beef. This step might have been difficult, but you did it!

In step 2, *substitute*, you found that other kinds of animal meats are just as tasty as beef. You further reduced the amount of beef you consumed weekly and ate other kinds of meat, like poultry and fish, instead. Did you ever think you'd be eating so little beef and so much "lighter" meat?

In step 3, *incorporate*, you began to discover the wonderful world of plant foods. Who would have thought that vegetables, whole grains, legumes, herbs, and fresh fruit could give your meals so much taste and be so satisfying—and with so many economic benefits! How wonderful! Perhaps you've already lost a few pounds in your Beef Busters journey. Another pleasantly surprising benefit.

And here you are at step 4, *eliminate*. You are ready to turn to a beef-free, low-fat, healthy diet that fights chronic disease with wonderfully satisfying plant foods. Recipes cover the range from one-pot wonders to enticing vegetable main courses with creative side dishes.

And who would have thought you would ever try tofu? In this chapter you'll find another delicious recipe using tofu. Remember that eating soy products might even help prolong your life. (See Chapter 9 for more on soy.)

RECIPES

Stuffed Mushrooms and Baked Corn Fritters

This meal is perfect for impressing a crowd. The mushrooms and the baked corn fritters are both low in fat, high in flavor, and make good snacks, buffet items, or components of an elegant sit-down dinner. Just double, triple, or quadruple the recipe for large groups. And sure, fritters are normally fried, but these maintain their shape with the help of mini-muffin tins. And because they are baked in the oven, they are much lower in fat than the traditional version.

STUFFED MUSHROOMS

SERVES 4

> *12 large white mushrooms*
> *1 teaspoon extra-virgin olive oil*
> *¼ cup minced yellow onion*
> *1 garlic clove, minced or put through a press*
> *½ small carrot, grated*
> *1 teaspoon crushed dried thyme*
> *1 tablespoon chopped fresh tarragon*
> *1 tablespoon freshly squeezed lemon juice*
> *⅓ cup fine dry whole-grain bread crumbs or crushed whole-grain croutons*
> *2 ounces poached or canned salmon, flaked*
> *1 tablespoon low-fat grated Parmesan cheese*

Preheat oven to 375°F. Spray a casserole just large enough to hold 12 mushroom caps with nonstick cooking spray.

Remove the stems from the mushroom caps. Put caps in the prepared casserole, cups facing up. Cut off the tough ends of the stems and discard. Finely chop the remaining stem parts.

Spray a medium nonstick skillet with cooking spray, then heat the oil over medium heat. Add the mushroom stems along with the onion, garlic, carrot, and thyme. Cook until the onion and mushrooms are soft, about 5 minutes. Remove from the heat and mix in the tarragon, lemon juice, bread crumbs, and salmon. Toss lightly until combined.

Spoon the mixture into the mushroom caps, stuffing each cap as full as possible. Tap down the stuffing over each mushroom with a spoon; when the caps are full, sprinkle the remaining onion mixture loosely over the tops of all the mushrooms. Sprinkle the cheese lightly and evenly over all the mushroom caps.

Bake 15 minutes, or until heated through. Allow to cool and set 5 minutes; then serve.

Nutritional information per serving: 108 calories, 3 grams total fat (1 gram saturated, 2 grams monounsaturated), 8 grams protein, 2 grams fiber, 2 milligrams iron, 9 milligrams cholesterol, 121 milligrams sodium

BAKED CORN FRITTERS

Serves 6

> *1 (15-ounce) can drained corn kernels or 1½ cups frozen and*
> *thawed kernels*
> *1 egg, beaten*
> *¼ cup unbleached all-purpose flour*
> *2 tablespoons cornmeal*
> *1 tablespoon honey*
> *1 teaspoon baking powder*
> *Dash salt*

Preheat oven to 375°F. Spray a 12-cup mini-muffin tin or a 6-cup medium muffin tin with nonstick cooking spray.

Combine all the ingredients in a medium bowl. Give the batter another stir (it tends to separate) and spoon it evenly into the prepared muffin cups, filling about ¾ of the way full. Scrape any remaining batter from the bowl and distribute evenly among the cups.

Bake 15 to 20 minutes for mini-muffins or 20 to 25 minutes for medium muffins, or until the fritters are puffed and golden brown. Allow to cool about 10 minutes before serving warm.

Nutritional information per serving: 107 calories, 2 grams total fat (0 gram saturated, 1 gram monounsaturated), 3 grams protein, 2 grams fiber, 1 milligram iron, 35 milligrams cholesterol, 335 milligrams sodium

NOTE: If you bake the fritters at the same time you're baking the mushrooms, the fritters may need to bake an extra 5 minutes or more. Watch for them to look puffed and golden.

Veggie Enchiladas with Spicy Rice

This Mexican-inspired meal is a lot lower in fat and calories than a typical dinner at a Mexican restaurant. You won't feel weighed down after this meal, but you will feel like you've enjoyed an exotic culinary experience.

VEGGIE ENCHILADAS

SERVES 4

> *8 (8-inch) flour tortillas*
> *½ teaspoon extra-virgin olive oil*
> *1 cup thinly sliced sweet onion*
> *½ cup thinly sliced mushrooms*
> *1 teaspoon all-purpose flour*
> *1 teaspoon chili powder*
> *1 medium tomato, cored and chopped*
> *1 (4-ounce) can chopped green chilies*
> *1 cup thinly sliced fresh spinach*
> *1 cup canned white beans, drained and rinsed*
> *2 tablespoons chopped fresh cilantro*
> *1 (10.75 ounce) can low-fat cream of mushroom soup*
> *1 cup (8 ounces) nonfat sour cream*
> *1 cup nonfat milk*
> *4 ounces fat-free Cheddar cheese*

Preheat the oven to 350°F. Spray a 12 by 8-inch casserole with nonstick cooking spray. Stack the tortillas and wrap them in foil. Put them in the oven while it is preheating.

Spray a large nonstick skillet with nonstick cooking spray and add the oil. Heat over medium-high heat. Add the onions and mushrooms; then sprinkle with the flour and chili powder. When the vegetables are soft but not brown, remove from the heat and add half of the tomato along with the green chilies, spinach, beans, and cilantro. Mix well.

Remove the tortillas from the oven and unwrap. Spoon one-eighth of the vegetable mixture onto each tortilla, roll them up, and place them in the prepared pan.

In a medium bowl, combine the soup, sour cream, and milk. Pour over the enchiladas. Sprinkle the remaining tomatoes over the top. Cover with foil and bake 30 minutes. Remove from the oven and immediately sprinkle the cheese over the top. Bake, uncovered, 5 minutes more. Allow the tortillas to stand 10 minutes before serving.

Nutritional information per serving: 590 calories, 13 grams total fat (3 grams saturated, 4 grams monounsaturated), 29 grams protein, 5 grams fiber, 5 milligrams iron, 5 milligrams cholesterol, 1378 milligrams sodium

NOTE: To reduce the sodium in this recipe, use reduced-sodium mushroom soup.

SPICY RICE

SERVES 4

> *2 cups raw brown or white rice*
> *1 (4-ounce) can chopped green chilies*
> *1 medium tomato, chopped*
> *2 green onions, finely chopped*
> *¼ cup tomato sauce*
> *1 ounce shredded nonfat Cheddar cheese*
> *½ teaspoon sweet paprika*
> *Dash cayenne*

Cook the rice according to the package's directions. While the rice is still hot, mix it with remaining ingredients and serve warm.

Nutritional information per serving: 380 calories, 3 grams total fat (1 gram saturated, 1 gram monounsaturated), 10 grams protein, 5 grams fiber, 2 milligrams iron, 1 milligram cholesterol, 204 milligrams sodium

ONE-POT SPINACH LASAGNA

This Italian-inspired dinner is filling and so delicious that you won't even notice it doesn't contain any meat! You may not have suspected that vegetarian food could be so good; but just try this meal, and you'll be a convert. Of course, that doesn't mean you have to eat vegetarian every night, but entrées like this can make vegetarian seem like a pretty pleasing prospect. Lasagna is typically a time-consuming recipe but this one-pot version is done in half the time—with half the fat!

SERVES 4

> *4 dried lasagna noodles*
> *1 tablespoon extra-virgin olive oil*
> *1 cup chopped onion*
> *1 garlic clove, minced or put through a press*
> *½ green bell pepper, chopped*
> *1 cup chopped fresh spinach*
> *1 cup sliced fresh mushrooms*
> *1 cup canned diced tomatoes*
> *1 cup tomato sauce*
> *1 teaspoon crushed dried basil*
> *1 teaspoon crushed dried oregano*
> *½ teaspoon crushed dried thyme*
> *8 ounces low-fat ricotta cheese*
> *4 teaspoons low-fat grated Parmesan cheese*

Break the lasagna noodles into bite-size pieces. Cook according to package's directions. Rinse quickly, drain, and put noodles into a bowl, and set aside.

Return the noodle pot to the stove over medium heat. Add the oil, onion, garlic, and bell pepper. Sauté until the vegetables are soft but not brown, about 10 minutes. Add the spinach, mushrooms, tomatoes, tomato sauce, basil, oregano, and thyme. Simmer 10 minutes, or until gently bubbling. Stir in the ricotta cheese and then add the noodles. Cook for a few more minutes, or until noodles are hot. Ladle the lasagna into individual bowls and sprinkle each serving with 1 teaspoon Parmesan cheese.

Nutritional information per serving: 248 calories, 8 grams total fat (3 grams saturated, 4 grams monounsaturated), 12 grams protein, 4 grams fiber, 3 milligrams iron, 17 milligrams cholesterol, 491 milligrams sodium

JAMBALAYA WITH SHRIMP AND TURKEY SAUSAGE

You can pretend you're heading down to the bayou for dinner when you make jambalaya. This version doesn't contain the traditional pieces of chicken, making room for more veggies. The shrimp and the turkey sausage give this dish plenty of meaty flavor without too much meat-based fat. Plus, the dish is really quick and easy to make if you use leftover rice and buy the shrimp already cooked. Just remember to choose sausage that contains 100 percent turkey or a mixture of turkey and chicken. Seafood sausage is a gourmet item that may be difficult to find, but it makes this dish extra special. Any sausage product you cook with must be beef-free.

SERVES 4

> *1 tablespoon extra-virgin olive oil*
> *1 medium yellow onion*
> *2 celery ribs, chopped*
> *1 medium green bell pepper, chopped*
> *1 medium red bell pepper, cut into 2-inch strips*
> *Pinch hot red pepper flakes*
> *¼ teaspoon freshly ground black pepper*
> *8 ounces cooked fresh shrimp*
> *4 ounces low-fat, low-sodium turkey sausage, sliced*
> *4 cups cooked yellow rice*
> *½ cup chicken broth*
> *Parsley, for garnish*

Heat the oil in a large nonstick skillet over medium heat. Add the onion, celery, and bell peppers; cook until tender. Stir in the red pepper flakes and black pepper. Add the shrimp and turkey sausage and mix into the vegetables. Heat for 5 minutes. Add the rice and broth. Mix well. Cook until heated through and the broth is absorbed.

To serve, mound on a platter and garnish with the parsley.

Nutritional information per serving: 437 calories, 10 grams total fat (2 grams saturated, 1 gram monounsaturated), 24 grams protein, 1 gram fiber, 5 milligrams iron, 132 milligrams cholesterol, 460 milligrams sodium

Creamy-Crunchy Egg Salad Sandwiches with Baked Carrot "Chips"

Creamy, crunchy comfort food, and low-fat, too. What else do you need for lunch? How about chips made from sweet, crunchy, antioxidant-rich carrots? Tasty.

CREAMY-CRUNCHY EGG SALAD SANDWICHES

SERVES 4

> *4 hard-boiled eggs*
> *1 tablespoon low-fat mayonnaise*
> *2 tablespoons nonfat plain yogurt*
> *1 tablespoon low-fat cottage cheese*
> *1 celery rib, chopped*
> *¼ medium green bell pepper, chopped*
> *1 tablespoon chopped pecans*
> *1 tablespoon pickle relish*
> *1 teaspoon dried dill*
> *8 slices whole-grain bread*
> *4 leaves buttercrunch lettuce*

Chop the eggs and place in a medium bowl. Mix in the mayonnaise, yogurt, and cottage cheese until combined. Add the celery, bell pepper, pecans, relish, and dill; stir to combine. Spread evenly on four slices of bread. Top each with a lettuce leaf and another slice of bread.

Nutritional information per serving: 239 calories, 8 grams total fat (2 grams saturated, 3 grams monounsaturated), 12 grams protein, 1 gram fiber, 3 milligrams iron, 187 milligrams cholesterol, 447 milligrams sodium

BAKED CARROT "CHIPS"

SERVES 4

> *4 carrots*
> *1 tablespoon (more or less, to taste) of a combination of your*
>   *favorite herbs and spices (see Note)*
> *Salt to taste (optional)*
> *Honey to taste (optional)*

Preheat the oven to 400°F. Spray a cookie sheet with butter-flavored or olive oil nonstick cooking spray.

Peel the carrots and slice into ¼-inch-thick disks. Arrange on the cookie sheet, spray with nonstick cooking spray, and sprinkle liberally with the herbs and spices. Bake 20 minutes or until the outside is golden and slightly crisp. Season with salt for savory chips or a little honey for sweet chips.

Nutritional information per serving (excluding extra salt and honey, for flavor): 8 calories, 0 gram total fat (0 gram saturated, 0 gram monounsaturated), 0 gram protein, 0.5 gram fiber, 0 milligram iron, 0 milligram cholesterol, 4 milligrams sodium

NOTE: Try one of these combinations: fresh or dried basil and garlic powder; fresh or dried tarragon and onion powder; dried orange peel and ground cinnamon; or curry powder and hot red pepper flakes.

TOFU SATAY WITH PEANUT SAUCE

Satay is a popular Indonesian dish served on skewers. It can work as a lunch or dinner. Don't let the sound of this dish turn you off. This dish provides the perfect setting for tofu because it has an intense flavor and highlights tofu's firm, meaty texture. The tofu in this recipe is sliced thin, well spiced, and cooked until crispy. Peanut sauce is the traditional accompaniment. To get a chewier texture, freeze the tofu and then thaw it before making this recipe.

SERVES 4

> ½ pound extra-firm tofu
> ⅓ cup Worcestershire sauce
> 2 tablespoons extra-crunchy peanut butter
> 1 tablespoon cider vinegar
> 1 tablespoon soy sauce
> 1 teaspoon freshly squeezed lime juice
> Pinch sugar
> Dash hot red pepper flakes, or to taste
> ¼ cup cornstarch or all-purpose flour

Slice the tofu into thin slices (about ¼-inch thick) so each slice is the length of the short end of the tofu block. Lay the strips on paper towels and cover with more paper towels. Press down to remove all the water. Place the strips in a small bowl and cover with the Worcestershire sauce. Set aside.

Put the peanut butter, vinegar, soy sauce, lime juice, sugar, and red pepper flakes in a small bowl. Mix vigorously until well combined. Set aside.

Remove the tofu from the Worcestershire sauce and place on fresh paper towels to drain. Spray a large nonstick saucepan with olive-oil cooking spray and heat over medium-high. Dredge the tofu strips in the cornstarch and place in saucepan. Sauté for about 5 minutes on each side. If you don't have room to cook them all at once, sauté the strips in two batches, respraying with cooking spray before second batch (remove the pan from heat before spraying). Place the strips on paper towels to cool. When cool enough to handle, thread each strip the long way onto a small wooden skewer.

To serve, spoon one-quarter of the peanut sauce onto each of four small plates, then arrange the skewers on top.

Nutritional information per serving: 154 calories, 8 grams total fat (1 gram saturated, 3 grams monounsaturated), 8 grams protein, 1 gram fiber, 3 milligrams iron, 0 milligram cholesterol, 519 milligrams sodium

HOLIDAY STUFFED SQUASH

This dish can make any holiday special, and it doesn't even contain turkey . . . or any meat at all. Perfect for vegetarians or anyone who wants to eat light during the traditionally calorie-heavy holidays, this meal is both comfortingly familiar and pleasingly different. Vegans can leave out the egg and use a little vegetable broth instead. Serve with mashed potatoes, salad, and fruit pie for a real holiday feast. This recipe is easily doubled for a larger crowd.

SERVES 4

> *2 medium butternut squash*
> *1 cup whole-grain croutons*
> *1 cup cooked brown rice*
> *½ medium onion, chopped*
> *½ cup raisins, soaked in a little orange juice or brandy*
> *2 tablespoons chopped walnuts*
> *1 teaspoon grated orange zest*
> *1 egg, beaten*

Preheat the oven to 400°F.

Cut each squash in half lengthwise. Scoop out the seeds and place the halves, cut side down, in one or two large baking pans. Prick the skins all over with a fork and bake about 30 minutes, or until tender when pierced with a fork. Remove from the oven and allow to cool about 15 minutes. Leave the oven on.

Turn over each squash half and scoop out most of the flesh from each shell, leaving the shells intact.

Put the pulp in a large bowl. Add the remaining ingredients. Mix well and stuff each shell with the dressing. Return to the oven and bake 15 to 20 minutes, or until stuffing is hot.

Nutritional information per serving: 311 calories, 6 grams total fat (1 gram saturated, 2 grams monounsaturated), 8 grams protein, 10 grams fiber, 3 milligrams iron, 54 milligrams cholesterol, 155 milligrams sodium

ARTICHOKE QUESADILLAS WITH CAPERS AND CHEESE

Elegant as an hors d'oeuvre and excellent as a light supper, these quesadillas are full of flavor.

SERVES 4

4 (8-inch) flour tortillas
1 cup chopped drained artichoke hearts
1 tablespoon capers
½ medium red bell pepper, thinly sliced
4 ounces low-fat Mozzarella cheese
1 tablespoon grated Parmesan cheese
Freshly ground black pepper, to taste

Preheat the oven to 400°F.

Spray the tortillas on both sides with nonstick cooking spray. Put them on a cookie sheet and bake for about 10 minutes, or until crisp and golden, flipping over once. Remove from the oven. Leave the oven on.

Top each tortilla evenly with the artichoke hearts, capers, and bell pepper. Sprinkle with the cheeses and black pepper. Bake for 10 minutes, or until the cheese is melted and just beginning to turn golden. To serve, cut each quesadilla into quarters with a pizza cutter.

Nutritional information per serving: 257 calories, 8 grams total fat (4 grams saturated, 3 grams monounsaturated), 14 grams protein, 0.5 gram fiber, 2 milligrams iron, 16 milligrams cholesterol, 617 milligrams sodium

SESAME CHICKEN SALAD

When you need a healthy lunch that will give you energy and make you feel great about yourself, try this salad.

SERVES 4

> *6 cups chopped mixed greens*
> *4 ounces cubed cooked chicken breast*
> *1 tablespoon sesame seeds*
> *1 hard-boiled egg, chopped*
> *1 cup chopped broccoli florets*
> *1 medium bell pepper, chopped*
> *2 carrots, shredded*
> *¼ cup white wine vinegar*
> *1 tablespoon freshly squeezed lemon juice*
> *1 tablespoon toasted sesame oil*
> *1 slice multi-grain bread, toasted and cubed*

Toss the greens, chicken, sesame seeds, egg, broccoli, bell pepper, and carrots in a large bowl. Combine the vinegar, lemon juice, and oil in a jar with a tightly fitting lid. Seal the jar and shake well. Pour over the salad and toss well. Sprinkle with the toast cubes and serve in large bowls.

Nutritional information per serving: 119 calories, 6 grams total fat (1 gram saturated, 2 grams monounsaturated), 9 grams protein, 3 grams fiber, 34 milligrams iron, 52 milligrams cholesterol, 70 milligrams sodium

TORTILLA CASSEROLE

Made with eggs, cheese, and your healthiest leftovers, this recipe makes a special brunch or a warm, comforting dinner. Easy to make, you can prepare the casserole the night before so it's ready to bake in the morning. It's even good at room temperature or cold, if you don't finish it all at one meal.

SERVES 6

6 (8-inch) flour tortillas

1 (4-ounce) can chopped green chilies

1 cup chopped mixed vegetables (see Note)

1 cup legumes (see Note)

6 ounces low-fat shredded Cheddar or Monterey jack cheese

4 eggs

1 cup buttermilk

1 cup skim milk

½ teaspoon sweet paprika

Preheat the oven to 375°F. Spray a 13 by 9-inch baking pan with nonstick cooking spray.

Tear three tortillas into bite-size pieces and cover the bottom of the pan. Spread half the green chilies over top. Cover with half the vegetables, half the legumes, and half the cheese. Repeat with another layer of tortillas, chilies, vegetables, legumes, and cheese.

In a medium bowl, beat the eggs. Stir in the buttermilk and skim milk until well blended. Pour the egg mixture over tortillas. Sprinkle with the paprika. *Can be made ahead up to this point: Cover with foil and refrigerate up to 12 hours before baking.* Bake 40 minutes, or until golden and puffed. To serve, cut into squares.

Nutritional information per serving: 380 calories, 18 grams total fat (8 grams saturated, 6 grams monounsaturated), 22 grams protein, 1 gram fiber, 4 milligrams iron, 170 milligrams cholesterol, 588 milligrams sodium

NOTE: For the vegetables, try a combination of grated carrots, chopped bell pepper, sliced mushrooms, chopped onion, sliced zucchini, or chopped tomato. For the legumes, try any cooked bean or even tofu cubes.

MONITOR YOUR PROGRESS—STEP 4

❏ I am incorporating legumes (and soy) into my meals at least four times a week.

❏ I am incorporating at least three servings of vegetables into my daily meals.

❏ I am incorporating at least two servings of fruits into my daily eating plan.

❏ I am incorporating at least six servings of whole grains into my daily eating plan.

❏ I am incorporating moderate amounts of unsalted nuts or seeds (or nut spreads) into my meals at least three times a week.

❏ I am incorporating fish sources of omega-3 fatty acids into my diet at least once (better, twice) a week.

❏ I have eliminated beef from my diet.

Congratulations! You've mastered the Beef Buster diet! Now, don't forget to get regular physical activity (after consulting your doctor and based on your individual fitness level) and to get plenty of rest and relaxation—important components of a healthy lifestyle!

Remember that the Beef Buster diet is a general guideline only. For an individually tailored diet, discuss nutrition with your primary care physician, or seek the help of a registered dietitian to ensure that you are meeting all of your particular nutritional requirements for a healthy existence.

Glossary

Amino acids. The building blocks of PROTEINS.

Antioxidants. Substances that reduce the formation of free radicals (which are believed to play a role in the development of many health problems, including heart disease and cancer).

Basal metabolic rate (BMR). The rate at which your body uses energy to fuel the basic activities that make life possible.

Body mass index (BMI). The standard weight-assessment tool among health-care professionals. Based on an individual's height and weight.

Bovine spongiform encephalopathy (BSE). Infectious, fatal brain-wasting disease that strikes cattle. People who eat beef from an infected cow can develop a similar disease called VARIANT CREUTZFELDT-JAKOB DISEASE. Belongs to a classification of diseases called transmittable spongiform encephalopathies (TSEs).

Calorie. A unit of measure commonly used to identify the energy values of foods and activities.

Campylobacteriosis. FOOD-BORNE ILLNESS caused by *Campylobacter* bacteria.

Carbohydrates. Primary form of energy from food; either simple (sugars) or complex (starch).

Carcinogen. Substance that causes cancer.

Cardiovascular disease. The accumulation of fatty deposits and plaque in the arteries (atherosclerosis) and stiffening of the arterial walls (arteriosclerosis) anywhere in the body, including the heart (CORONARY HEART DISEASE) and brain (CEREBROVASCULAR DISEASE).

Carnivorous. Meat eating.

Carotenoids. PHYTOCHEMICALS believed to enhance immunity and inhibit the growth of cancer cells. Found in brightly colored vegetables, such as carrots and sweet potatoes.

Cerebrovascular disease. Blockage from fatty deposits and hardening of the arteries that supply the brain; stroke can be the consequence.

Cholesterol, blood. The levels of cholesterol in the bloodstream; not the same as DIETARY CHOLESTEROL.

Cholesterol, dietary. The cholesterol we eat; found only in animal-based foods.

Coronary heart disease (CHD). Blockage from fatty deposits in the arteries that supply the heart; heart attack can be the consequence.

Creutzfeldt-Jakob Disease (CJD). Rare, fatal disease that attacks and destroys brain tissue. Most cases occur randomly; a small percentage are familial (run in certain families). Does not appear to be contagious and is *not* the same as VARIANT CREUTZFELDT-JAKOB DISEASE (vCJD), associated with eating beef from cows that have BSE.

Daidzein. An isoflavonoid found in soybeans that appears to slow and possibly prevent the growth of certain cancers as well as to enhance the body's immune response.

Diabetes mellitus. Illness in which the pancreas stops producing insulin (type 1 or juvenile onset) or in which the body can no longer use insulin efficiently (type 2 or adult onset).

Digestion. Process of breaking food down into the nutrients the body needs.

Disaccharide. A simple sugar that can be further broken down into two MONOSACCHARIDE molecules, such as sucrose (common table sugar).

Embolus. A dislodged piece of arterial plaque that enters the bloodstream and can cause heart attack or stroke by blocking an artery.

Enteritis. Inflammation of the intestinal tract, often caused by food-borne PATHOGENS.

Escherichia coli **O157:H7.** Strain of bacteria that, when it contaminates beef and other foods, can cause serious illness and even death; abbreviated as *E. coli*.

Essential. Substances the body must obtain through dietary sources and cannot manufacture from other substances, such as essential AMINO ACIDS and essential fatty acids.

Fad diet. Diet that claims rapid weight loss through following a specific regimen; such diets cycle rapidly in and out of popularity. Most are ineffective for consistent, long-term weight loss.

Fat, monounsaturated. Fatty acid with one less than a full complement of hydrogen molecules. Found in olive oil, canola oil, nuts, and seeds. Believed to raise "good" BLOOD CHOLESTEROL levels.

Fat, polyunsaturated. Fatty acid with multiple missing hydrogen molecules in its chemical chain. Liquid or soft at room temperature and includes some vegetable oils, such as corn and safflower oil. Believed to have no effect on BLOOD CHOLESTEROL levels.

Fat, saturated. Fatty acid that contains a full complement of hydrogen molecules. Found mostly in animal-based foods, such as fatty meats and butter. Stays solid at room temperature. Raises "bad" BLOOD CHOLESTEROL levels, increasing the risk for heart disease.

Fat-burning foods. Promotional hype for fad diets. There are no foods that burn fat.

Fiber, insoluble. Fiber the body cannot digest; promotes a healthy digestive tract. Found in wheat bran.

Fiber, soluble. Fiber that dissolves into substances and helps the body eliminate cholesterol. Found in oats and beans.

Fixed risk. A risk factor that you cannot change, such as heredity; also called an absolute risk.

Flavonoids. A large class of PHYTOCHEMICALS that appear to slow or even prevent cancer and heart disease.

Food-borne illness. Infection that results from foods contaminated by PATHOGENS such as bacteria and parasites.

Foot and mouth disease (FMD). Highly infectious viral infection that causes sores and blisters on the mouths and feet of animals with split hooves. Not known to infect humans.

Genestein. An isoflavonoid found in soybeans that appears to slow and possibly prevent the growth of certain cancers as well as to enhance the body's immune response.

Glycogen. Energy stores, in the form of converted glucose, in the body's muscle tissues and liver.

Grain, refined. Food products made from just the endosperm of the grain.

Grain, whole. Food products that include all edible parts of the grain (bran, endosperm, and germ).

Hazard Analysis and Critical Control Point (HACCP). U.S. DEPARTMENT OF AGRICULTURE preventive approach to reducing the incidence of violations of food regulations and safe slaughter practices.

Healthy weight. Medically defined as a BODY MASS INDEX between 18 and 24.9; optimal for health.

Heterocyclic amines (HCAs). MUTAGENS that form when meat cooks, especially at high temperatures. Believed to cause certain kinds of cancer.

High density lipoprotein (HDL). "Good" BLOOD CHOLESTEROL.

Hypertension. Clinical term for high blood pressure.

Immune system disorder. Any of numerous forms of disease in which the immune system, the body system that prevents and fights infection, is not functioning properly.

Irradiation. Exposing food products to gamma radiation to kill PATHOGENS; approved for limited and specific uses in the United States (irradiated foods must prominently labeled as such).

Isoflavones. FLAVONOIDS (PHYTOCHEMICALS) found abundantly in soybeans that appear effective in preventing some forms of cancer, such as breast cancer and prostate cancer.

Ketone bodies. Chemical substances produced when the body metabolizes fat for energy.

Ketosis. Abnormally high level of KETONE BODIES in the bloodstream and urine, indicating that the body has slowed its insulin production.

Listeriosis. FOOD-BORNE ILLNESS caused by *Listeria monocytogenes* bacteria.

Low density lipoprotein (LDL). "Bad" BLOOD CHOLESTEROL.

Lutein. A powerful ANTIOXIDANT that appears to prevent age-related macular degeneration, a leading cause of blindness. Found in foods such as spinach and collard greens.

Lycopenes. A CAROTENOID (PHYTOCHEMICAL) believed to prevent and fight certain cancers. Found in foods such as tomatoes and watermelon.

Meat Inspection Act of 1906. U.S. legislation requiring federal inspection of slaughterhouses and beef products.

Minerals. Chemicals found in foods that your body needs for health, such as calcium and iron.

Miso. A fermented paste made from soybeans that has the consistency of peanut butter and a mild flavor.

Monosaccharide. Simplest form of sugar that cannot be further broken down, such as glucose and fructose.

Mutable risk. A risk factor that you can change, such as diet or smoking; also called a relative risk.

Mutagen. A changed chemical substance; as meat cooks, mutagens form. May cause diseases, such as cancer.

Obesity. Medically defined as a BODY MASS INDEX higher than 30. Linked to various health conditions and medical problems.

Omega-3 fatty acid. A form of dietary fat found in some fish (such as salmon, tuna, and mackerel), flaxseed, and walnuts. Believed to help reduce the risk for heart disease.

Organically grown foods. Foods that meet U.S. standards restricting the use of chemicals during growth and processing; does not mean the foods are chemical free.

Osteoporosis. Disease in which the body draws calcium from the bones, leaving the bones weakened; most common in women after menopause.

Overweight. Medically defined as a BODY MASS INDEX between 25 and 29.9; associated with an increased risk of health problems.

Pathogen. Agent capable of causing illness or disease, such as bacteria and viruses.

Phytochemicals. Substances found uniquely in plants that appear to protect the body from disease, such as cancer and heart disease.

Phytoestrogens. Plant-based estrogen chemicals abundant in foods such as soybeans.

Plaque. Fatty deposits that accumulate along the walls of the arteries.

Prion. PROTEIN-like structure that lacks a nucleus. One type is believed to be the agent responsible for causing BSE in cows and VARIANT CREUTZFELDT-JAKOB DISEASE in people.

Protein. Dietary substance that provides the body with AMINO ACIDS, from which cells manufacture the structures they need to function. A complete dietary protein supplies all nine ESSENTIAL amino acids that the human body requires.

Pure Food and Drug Act. U.S. federal legislation, passed in 1906, making it illegal to mislabel or adulterate food and drug products.

Recommended Dietary Allowance (RDA). The amount of a particular nutrient required to meet the daily needs of an average, healthy individual.

Salmonellosis. FOOD-BORNE ILLNESS caused by *Salmonella* bacteria.

Sedentary. Physically inactive.

Serving size. The amount of food consumed at one time; the basis on which nutritional information is calculated. Health experts generally recommend smaller serving sizes than many Americans typically eat.

Sulforaphanes. Powerful cancer-fighting PHYTOCHEMICALS found in cruciferous vegetables, such as broccoli and cabbage.

Tempeh. A firm cake made from a fermented mixture of soybeans and grain; has a nutty flavor.

Textured soy protein (TSP). Products made from soy available in many forms, including some that emulate burgers, hot dogs, and lunch meats.

Thrombus. Blood clot that breaks free and enters the bloodstream, where it can cause heart attack or stroke by blocking an artery.

Tofu. A versatile, mild-flavored soy product made from soybean curds, much as cheese is made from milk.

Trans fatty acids. Fat structure created when a hydrogen molecule is artificially added to an otherwise UNSATURATED FAT to extend the product's shelf life. Believed to increase the risk for heart disease as much as SATURATED FATS.

U.S. Department of Agriculture (USDA). Federal agency responsible for overseeing farming and ranching operations in the United States.

Variant Creutzfeldt-Jakob disease (vCJD). The form of fatal brain-wasting disease that affects people who eat beef from cows with BSE.

Vegan. Eating strictly fruits, vegetables, grains, legumes, nuts, and seeds with no animal-based or dairy products.

Vegetarian. Eating predominantly fruits, vegetables, grains, legumes, nuts, and seeds; many vegetarians also occasionally eat eggs and dairy products.

Vitamins. Substances found in foods that the body needs for metabolism.

Yo-yo dieting. Unhealthy cycle of losing weight, usually rapidly, and then regaining the lost weight and usually more.

Resources

Here's where to find more information on the topics covered in this book.

General Nutrition

Duyff, Roberta Larson. *The American Dietetic Association's Complete Food and Nutrition Guide.* Minneapolis: Chronimed Publishing, 1998.

A book that provides comprehensive information about foods and nutrition, including fitness tips and weight-management strategies.

www.eatright.org

The Web site for the American Dietetic Association (ADA) features nutrition and lifestyle information. Includes a national dietitian locator service ("Find a Dietitian").

www.usda.gov

The U.S. Department of Agriculture's Web site provides extensive and diverse information about all aspects of nutrition and diet, including the current version of *Dietary Guidelines for Americans.* There are special sections that cover nutritional health issues for seniors, women, and children.

www.cfsan.fda.gov

The Web site for the U.S. Center for Food Safety and Applied Nutrition (a division of the Food and Drug Administration) provides a wide range of information about safe food-handling practices and general nutrition.

Maintaining Health and Preventing Disease through Lifestyle

www.americanheart.org

The Web site for the American Heart Association provides an abundance of information about heart disease and what steps you can take to reduce your risks.

www.cancer.org

The American Cancer Society's Web site provides extensive information about all forms of cancer. Includes suggestions for lifestyle changes to reduce your risks for getting cancer. Also provides information about different kinds of treatment.

www.diabetes.org

The American Diabetes Association's Web site provides general information about diabetes as well as nutrition and lifestyle recommendations.

Food-Borne Illness and Food-Related Health Issues

www.fda.gov

The Web site for the U.S. Food and Drug Administration (FDA) features information about the products it regulates, new product approvals, recalls, and health topics in the news. The site also includes background fact sheets and the latest action reports about food-borne illnesses, including bovine spongiform encephalopathy (BSE) and variant Creutzfeldt-Jakob disease (vCJD).

www.cdc.gov

The Web site for the Centers for Disease Control and Prevention (CDC) provides summary as well as comprehensive information about the kinds of food-borne illnesses that infect Americans, infection rates, preventive measures, and risks. The site also provides regularly updated guidelines and advisories for travelers about bovine spongiform encephalopathy (BSE).

www.foodsafety.gov

A Web site sponsored jointly by a number of U.S. federal government agencies that functions as a gateway to other Web sites that provide food safety information.

www.fsis.usda.gov

The Web site for the U.S. Department of Agriculture's Food Safety and Inspection Service (FSIS) features news and information about food safety issues and food-borne illnesses.

www.who.int

The Web site for the World Health Organization (WHO) has background information, reports, and recommended precautions related to bovine spongiform encephalopathy (BSE) and variant Creutzfeldt-Jakob disease (vCJD).

www.maff.gov.uk/animalh/bse/

Web page from the U.K. Department of Environment, Food and Rural Affairs (DEFRA) that features in-depth information about bovine spongiform encephalopathy (BSE) and variant Creutzfeldt-Jakob disease (vCJD).

www.humanbse.org.uk

The families and friends of victims of variant Creutzfeldt-Jakob disease (vCJD) operate this Web site, which provides information about the disease, a support network for those who have family members or friends with vCJD, and resources for additional information.

www.cjdfoundation.org

The Web site for the Creutzfeldt-Jakob Disease Foundation provides comprehensive information about CJD, vCJD, and bovine spongiform encephalopathy (BSE).

www.sparc.airtime.co.uk/bse

A Web site that features extensive links to information and resources related to bovine spongiform encephalopathy (BSE) and variant Creutzfeldt-Jakob disease (vCJD).

www.europa.eu.int

The Web site for the European Union; run a search for "BSE" or "vCJD" to obtain a list of available articles and reports about the diseases.

U.S. Department of Agriculture Meat and Poultry Hotline

In the United States, call this hotline at 800-535-4555 (or TTY for the hearing-impaired at 800-256-7072) with questions or for safe meat handling and recall information.

Index

About the Authors

Marissa Cloutier, M.S., R.D., is a registered dietician with a Master of Science in human nutrition and metabolism from Boston University. She is a food and nutrition instructor at Briarwood College in Southington, CT. She is the author, with Eve Adamson, of *The Mediterranean Diet*, and has written articles for the *Tufts University Health & Nutrition Newsletter* and for a Boston University "healthy aging" Web site. She trained at The Beth Israel Hospital in Boston, a primary teaching hospital of the Harvard University School of Medicine, and was a clinical dietitian at the Faulkner Hospital in Boston, a teaching hospital of the Tufts University School of Medicine. She is a member of the American Dietetic Association, the Connecticut Dietetic Association, and the American Medical Writers Association. Marissa and her family enjoy the many wonderful flavors and health benefits of a beef-free, primarily vegetarian, Beef Buster diet. Marissa currently lives in Connecticut.

Deborah S. Romaine has authored, co-authored, or contributed to 14 books, including *Syndrome X: Managing Insulin Resistance*, with Jennifer B. Marks, M.D., and *The Complete Idiot's Guide to Healing Back Pain*, with Dawn E. DeWitt, M.D. She has published more than 350 articles. She specializes in writing about health and lifestyle topics, and collaborated with Marissa on the health and nutrition chapters of *Beef Busters*. Deborah has a Master of Arts degree in English/Creative Writing from the University of Washington. Although Deborah already eats a diet low in fat and cholesterol, after researching this book she doubts she'll ever be tempted to bring beef back as a mainstay on the family table. She lives with her family in Washington State's Puget Sound area.

Eve Adamson has authored or co-authored 14 books, including *The Mediterranean Diet*, with Marissa Cloutier, M.S., R.D., and *The Complete Idiot's Guide to Zen Living*, with Gary McClain, Ph.D. She has a Master of Fine Arts degree in creative writing from the University of Florida. Eve collaborated with Marissa on the recipes and menu planner for *Beef Busters*. Although never crazy about beef to begin with, working on this book has helped Eve and her family to swear off beef completely. "Even if I can be almost positive a given piece of meat is safe to eat, there are so many other implications for me: What if this is the first bad batch and they discover it because my family gets sick? Is the momentary pleasure of a burger worth the health risk, from food-borne contamination, from saturated fat, or from the unknown danger of mad cow disease? Do I want to contribute to the consumption of animals, when I'm not comfortable with the way most of those animals are kept and killed? Do I want to feel healthier, have more energy, and feel more in harmony with the world around me? These days, I'm much more likely to make my decision based on questions like these. I find the diversity in flavor, texture, color, and nutritional value of plant foods much more interesting and conducive to creativity in the kitchen." Eve lives in Iowa City with her two sons.

About the Contributors

Foreword writer **Nancy A. Tarantino, M.S.,** received a Bachelor of Science degree in biology from West Virginia Wesleyan College and a Master of Science degree in health administration from New Jersey City University. She is licensed by the N.J. Department of Health and Senior Services as a Registered Environmental Health Specialist and Health Officer, and has worked as a health inspector for the Hoboken, New Jersey Health Department since 1989.

Technical editor **Glenn Rothfeld, M.D., M.Ac.,** served as a clinical fellow at Harvard University School of Medicine after his training in family medicine. He is trained in nutritional and herbal medicine and has a Master's degree in acupuncture. Medical director for WholeHealth New England, Dr. Rothfeld is also clinical assistant professor of community health and family health at Tufts University School of Medicine. Dr. Rothfeld is the author several books, most recently *The Acupuncture Response.*

In addition to her online business at *www.onlinedietician.net,* **Linda Horning, R.D.,** enjoys a career in community nutrition, both as a WIC nutritionist for the USDA Supplemental Nutrition Program for Women, Infants, and Children, and as a Head Start nutrition coordinator. More recently, her work providing nutritional analyses of menus, including those in *Beef Busters*, has enabled Linda to see how easy it is to plan healthy meals when the focus is on fruits and vegetables. Plant-based diets contain all of the cancer and heart disease fighting properties, while leaving out those that lead to weight gain and poor nutrition. Now, when over nutrition is more of a concern than under nutrition, Linda supports efforts that help us curb our appetite for beef.